Small Board-and-Care Homes ☐

☐ # Small
Board-and-Care
Homes

Residential Care in Transition

**Leslie A. Morgan,
J. Kevin Eckert, and
Stephanie M. Lyon**

The Johns Hopkins University Press
Baltimore and London

© 1995 The Johns Hopkins University Press
All rights reserved. Published 1995
Printed in the United States of America on acid-free paper
04 03 02 01 00 99 98 97 96 95   5 4 3 2 1

The Johns Hopkins University Press
2715 North Charles Street
Baltimore, Maryland 21218-4319
The Johns Hopkins Press Ltd., London

Library of Congress Cataloging-in-Publication Data will be found
at the end of this book.
A catalog record for this book is available from the British Library.

ISBN 0-8018-4996-9

Contents □

ACKNOWLEDGMENTS   vii

1 The Board-and-Care Industry in American Society   1

2 The Board-and-Care Environment   24

3 The Economics of Small Board-and-Care Homes   51

4 Operators of the Homes   86

5 The Residents   118

6 Social Supports and Relationships in the Homes   149

7 The Future of Small Board-and-Care Homes   182

APPENDIX: DETAILS OF THE RESEARCH   207

REFERENCES   219

INDEX   231

Acknowledgments □

□ THE COMPLETION of a major research study, and especially two major research studies, emphasizes to those involved the very real contributions of a variety of persons on many levels. Our initial thanks must go to the National Institute on Aging of NIH for providing the funding that enabled us to carry out these projects in the Cleveland and Baltimore metropolitan areas. While NIA is in no way responsible for our results or conclusions, including any errors, they enabled a vigorous and rewarding collection of data on small board-and-care homes. A special word of thanks goes to Marcia Ory of NIA, who provided us with support and guidance throughout these projects.

A second round of appreciation goes to the research teams in the two research cities. In Cleveland, Drs. Marie Haug and Eva Kahana were co-principal investigators on the project, providing valuable insight on the design of the study. Dr. Kevan Namazi served as the project director, skillfully coordinating the construction of the survey instruments, data collection, and initial data analyses. Drs. Robert Rubinstein and Sally Reisacher consulted on sample and survey development. The Boarding Home Advocacy Program of Cleveland played a major role in generating the sample of small homes. Finally, Eleanor Warner, Esq., provided guidance on the public policy dimensions of our work. All of these individuals deserve special credit and thanks.

In Baltimore, our hearty thanks go to an excellent team of interviewers and health evaluators, including Julia B. Anderson, Donna Cox, Gale DeHaven, Mary Pilcher, and Mara K. Skruch. Three of these five completed the Ph.D. while work on this research was under way, with two drawing dissertations from the studies of small board-and-care homes. They were more than data gatherers, serving also as key members of the team in the development of conceptual issues and analytic frameworks. The research process was much improved by their hard work and insights.

Other key team members in Baltimore included Drs. Jay Sokolovsky and Maria Vesperi, whose qualitative data collection enriched the process, and Dr. Derek Gill, for in-depth work on economic operations of homes in Baltimore. Our colleagues who assisted us as consultants in Baltimore were Dr. Susan Sherman and Dr. Steven Zarit. We also appreciate the efforts of Derek Gill as departmental chair and Dean Arthur Pittenger, who provided us both the time and the on-site support required for our work. Patricia Richardson provided typing support, and Mary Pat Armstrong and Sue Hahn provided administrative support.

A third and very important round of appreciation goes to the operators and residents of board-and-care homes in Cleveland and Baltimore. They gave generously of their time and thoughts and endured repeated, sometimes lengthy visits without always being sure of our purposes. Many of the operators are remarkably patient and giving people, and they deserve a lot more appreciation than they seem to get from society.

Finally, we would like to thank our respective spouses, Daniel McClain, Ellen Eckert, and Warren Lyon, for understanding when we had Saturday meetings and weekend or evening writing, analysis, and editing demands to work on "the book."

Small Board-and-Care Homes □

1 □ The Board-and-Care Industry in American Society

Why Is Board-and-Care an Issue?

THE CURRENT crisis surrounding the health and long-term care systems has given new life to the search for home- and community-based alternatives to traditional nursing home care. Concerns about the containment of cost, the quality of care, and the provision of community-based alternatives are part of the contemporary debate on long-term care for dependent populations of all types. These concerns have been spurred by biomedical and technological advances that have permitted larger numbers of persons to survive to ages when physical impairment and chronic illness become likely to limit independent living (Dunlop 1979).

Although most of the elderly are not disabled, for those who survive beyond age eighty-five, the chance of being limited in activity and in need of health and social services is increased (Senate 1988). Demographic changes are most dramatic among the "oldest old," who will constitute over 25 percent of those over sixty-five by the year 2050 (ibid.). The techniques for prolonging life have not been accompanied by advances in the treatment of chronic diseases that undermine the ability to live independently (Johnson and Grant 1985). The consequence is the emergence of a larger population of older persons, who, as they age, will require supportive residential settings and services (Dobkin 1989). This need will be especially acute for those persons with limited financial and social resources for care, since society cannot rely on a profit-motivated marketplace to provide low-cost alternatives (Ehrlich 1986; McCoy and Conley 1990; Senate 1988).

Board-and-care homes are one community-based option being increasingly identified as a critical, yet largely untapped, resource for long-term care in the United States (Dobkin 1989). Long-term care constitutes a set of health, personal care, and social services delivered over time to persons with some degree of functional incapacity (Kane and Kane 1987). Only recently have researchers begun to examine the range of long-term care options and alternatives within the middle ground between institutional and home care. As noted by Rubinstein (1995), research on this middle range includes such alternatives as sheltered housing (Butler, Oldman, and Greve 1983; Sherwood et al. 1981); domiciliary care (Sherwood, Morris, and Sherwood 1986); certified adult residential environments; intermediate-care housing (Brody 1975); adult foster care (McCoin 1983; Sherman and Newman 1988); assisted living (Regnier, Hamilton, and Yatabe 1991; Kane, Wilson, and Clemmer 1993); "alternative modes of living" (Eckert and Murrey 1984); the small congregate home (Murray 1988); congregate and other planned housing (Mollica and Ryther 1987; Kaye and Monk 1991); shared housing (Jaffee 1989; Streib, Folts, and Hilker 1984); and single-room occupancy hotels (Eckert 1980; Felton, Lehman, and Adler 1981; Overbo, Minkler, and Liljestrand 1991).

Board-and-care is a generic term used to describe a range of noninstitutional residential care arrangements (Conley 1989), including many of the above titles under its umbrella. Board-and-care homes range from large to small and from intimate to institutional (Mor, Sherwood, and Gutkin 1986; House 1989), with confusing terminology and problems in distinguishing such homes from other places offering care without medical treatment (McCoy and Conley 1990; Stone and Newcomer 1986).

In general, board-and-care homes house vulnerable adult populations who often lack key resources, serving populations that are poor, have inadequate kin and other social supports, and who suffer from long-term disabilities, mental illness, mental retardation, and chronic physical conditions (Eckert and Lyon 1991; McCoin 1983; Sherman and Newman 1988). Older people constitute an estimated 40 to 60 percent of the board-and-care population, with the largest category of residents being older, functionally impaired women (Dobkin 1989).

The board-and-care industry is controversial, since much of what is known about it comes variously from negative and sensational media coverage of selected tragedies and abuses, from the reports of regulators, who tend to see only the worst homes, or from public hearings that emphasize the negative aspects of board-and-care homes to elevate them as an issue requiring legislative action. Widely publicized abuses and tragedies in unregulated board-and-care homes over the past two decades have spurred the federal government and many state governments to increase attempts to regulate the industry (Hawes et al. 1993; Moon 1989). More recently, board-and-care homes have received renewed attention as policymakers search for cost-effective, community-based alternatives to expensive nursing home care (Dittmar 1989; Dobkin 1989). Market forces, influenced by regulations governing Medicaid funding, are driving nursing homes in the direction of limiting admission to those patients who require more intensive levels of care (Doty 1993). Although board-and-care homes can meet the needs of many of the less-impaired residents, funding has been slow to follow the need.

In the future, society's emphasis on policies favoring institutional settings for the care of the elderly and other dependent adults is likely to change (Doty 1993). Demographic trends will require the development and funding of home- and community-based care options for the elderly and disabled unable to live independently but not in need of skilled nursing care. As a result of most people's preference to remain in the community and, if possible, in their own homes (Doty 1993; Kane and Kane 1987), policies and funding may favor more flexible forms of long-term care in noninstitutional housing with supportive services. Board-and-care homes could be expanded to fill the growing gap in the continuum of care from independence in one's home to institutionalization (Hawes et al. 1993). As our findings show, small board-and-care homes occupy an important and distinctive niche in the long-term care continuum.

This book reports on the findings of empirical studies of small board-and-care homes in two metropolitan areas: Cleveland, Ohio, and Baltimore, Maryland. The remainder of this chapter focuses on the conceptual and methodological approaches used to study small board-and-care homes in the two areas. Ambiguity surrounding the definition of what constitutes board and care, its financing, and regulation provides a background for discussion of its marginal status in the long-term care continuum. The marginal status of small board-and-care homes further contributes to pressures and problems for those who operate and live in the homes and those who are responsible for protecting the dependent population they house.

Defining Board-and-Care

Varied and Confused Definitions

Board-and-care homes are nonmedical, community-based residences for unrelated dependent adults requiring in-home care and services. They range from very small, community-based homes to larger, more institutional facilities. Board-and-care homes typically provide shelter (room), meals (board), twenty-four-hour supervision, housekeeping, laundry, personal care, recreation, and other services to residents.

Legal definitions of *board* and *care* depend on local, state, and national statutes and are related to the health and welfare auspices under which homes are monitored. What is called *adult foster care* in one jurisdiction and funded primarily by Supplemental Security Income (SSI) (Center for the

Study of Social Policy [CSSP] 1988) may, for example, be referred to elsewhere as *sheltered housing*.

Estimates on the number of board-and-care homes nationally depend on how you define them. A 1987 industry survey identified about 563,000 board-and-care beds in 41,000 licensed homes nationally (GAO 1989). A more recent GAO study found some 75,000 licensed and unlicensed homes serving a million persons, including a half million disabled elders (GAO 1992). McCoy and Conley (1990, 147) estimated that there are nearly 70,000 licensed and unlicensed board-and-care homes housing nearly a million elders and others and that "3.2 million are estimated to be at immediate risk of board and care placement."

Small, Familial Homes

Lawton (1981) defined small board-and-care homes as single-family households with no more than four nonrelatives as paying residents. Other authors have attempted to define the social dimensions of these settings. They specify as highly desirable the creation of an atmosphere in which residents are treated as family members, participating in normal life activities (Sherman and Newman 1977; Silverstone 1978). The concept of a familylike primary group was highlighted as a key factor differentiating foster care from "mere boarding homes" (Sherman and Newman 1977). In reference to foster family arrangements, Silverstone (1978) suggested that they should offer older adults in need of care—over and above basic essentials—relatively permanent primary group relations wherein their individualized, affectional, and unpredictable needs are met. In such a context the resident was expected to reciprocate by trying to meet these needs for other primary group members. The foster family potentially offered closer links to the community of which the foster family was a part and independence from the conforming tendencies of institutional populations. Lawton (1981) noted that there was wide variation in the type and quality of foster homes and cautioned against assuming that security, social, and privacy needs were uniformly met in them.

The definition of small board-and-care homes used in the studies reported here focuses on the number of persons being cared for in the home, rather than the physical size of the residence, although the two factors are somewhat related. In fact, the sizes of homes measured in this client-based way varied from zero to twenty-three in Cleveland, where no regulation was in effect at the time of the study, and from one to fifteen in the Baltimore study, where homes of four or more residents were purportedly licensed at the start of the study.

Some of the larger homes in Maryland operated under special agreements between the counties and the state health department, permitting local oversight without licensure. The sizes and configurations of the homes in the two samples differed somewhat, in part as a function of differing regulatory circumstances in the two states. Since the time data were collected, Ohio has instituted a regulatory scheme that has apparently reduced the number of smaller homes, while increasing larger homes and forcing some small homes to go out of business or "underground" (Applebaum and Ritchey 1992). Maryland also has instituted a "registration" process for homes caring for two to four residents and has been granting permits to these homes since late 1991.

In reviewing other studies on the board-and-care industry, it appeared that both size and the coresidence of the operator differentiated between the small, familial types of homes we were most interested in studying and larger, more institutional, "staffed" homes that resembled more "medicalized" and larger-scale forms of care such as congregate homes or nursing homes. Dittmar (1989) found that smaller homes were more likely to have live-in staff and reflect the "mom-and-pop" model of operation. Larger homes were "staffed" from the outside and were more likely to be regulated by the state and run by business interests. To address this diversity and to create a more coherent grouping of homes, we restricted the samples for this book to homes that (1) housed eight or fewer residents at the time they were studied and (2) had a coresiding operator.

Our restrictions removed the larger homes from both samples (five homes in Baltimore, thirty-one homes in Cleveland) and the few additional homes (one in Baltimore, one in Cleveland) where the operator did not appear to reside with her clients. It was reassuring to see that in most instances the two criteria overlapped, so that the larger homes were also those least likely to have the operator in residence.

This resulted in an initial sample of 103 homes in Baltimore. Collecting information from operators on the residents from these homes over all four interviews resulted in a sample of 342 Baltimore residents for whom selected information was available. Similarly, the Cleveland samples were reduced to 146 homes and 217 residents, since residents in the eliminated homes were also excluded from the study. These reduced samples provided the basis for a more parsimonious description of the circumstances within small board-and-care homes in the two urban areas.

Variation among Small Homes

Additional variables important to consider in differentiating board-and-care settings include the fees paid for care, the race of the caregivers, and participation in the Project HOME regulatory/subsidy program in Baltimore. These variables provide contrasts among the homes throughout this book.

As noted above, smaller-size homes may provide an environment more conducive to the development of one-to-one relationships, individualized care, or a familylike atmosphere (Sherman and Newman 1988). Thus, our analysis examines the differences between small board-and-care homes housing one to three residents and those with four to eight residents.

The fees charged by operators are another important factor to consider in assuring the survival and quality of small board-and-care homes (Mor, Sherwood, and Gutkin 1986; Stone and Newcomer 1986). Differences among small board-and-care homes were examined on the basis of whether an operator charged residents "low" or "high" fees compared with the average in that location.

Cultural variations based on race may account for differences within the social milieu of small board-and-care homes. For example, African American operators may be more likely than white operators to promote values that encourage a more familylike atmosphere to develop in the home (Skruch 1993). Racial differences also may affect the levels of burden expressed by operators in caring for dependent adults (Hinrichsen and Ramirez 1992). Thus, analysis based on whether the operator was black or white is the third element for consideration in each chapter.

Finally, the significance of program auspices was considered by comparing homes in Baltimore that participated in Project HOME, a regulatory program described in somewhat greater detail later in this chapter, with those that did not.

A Brief History of Board-and-Care

McCoin (1983) provided a comprehensive history of adult foster care from its earliest origins in Western culture through the 1970s. Care for dependent adults in the homes of unrelated individuals is documented back to the fourteenth century in Gheel, Belgium, where adults with emotional problems were housed in private homes under the auspices of the Catholic Church. The practice was subsequently established in Scotland in the mid– nineteenth century and spread to the United States. The board-and-care industry may have also existed elsewhere without documentation as an underground, grass-roots community strategy for dealing with dependent and displaced persons.

In 1855 Massachusetts became the first state to adopt a policy to provide adult foster care to mental patients (McCoin 1983). Although other states were slow to follow, regulations governing housing for dependent adult populations (deinstitutionalized mentally ill, mentally retarded, physically disabled, dependent elderly) now exist, in various forms, in all states.

Sherman and Newman (1988) assert that board-and-care homes developed from two sources: (1) family-based and other care options for the mentally ill and (2) boarding homes and almshouses for the poor elderly. Since the early nineteenth century, the mentally ill were separated from society and cared for in asylums, institutions typically hidden from the mainstream of community life (Goffman 1961). By the middle of the nineteenth century, developments in the field of mental health reshaped treatment modalities for the mentally ill. Living in smaller groups or cottages within an institutional setting became common, as did farmlike settings, where the farm work could be performed by patients. In the twentieth century, with advances in treatment, institutional settings became increasingly medicalized; "mental hospitals" became the predominant method for treating the mentally ill (House 1989).

Advances in the treatment of mental illness in the 1950s, particularly the development of ataractic and antidepressive drugs, enabled many mentally ill persons who previously would have been institutionalized to live in the community. These advances, coupled with the advent of Medicaid, the federal-state program for the very poor, created a motivation for states to discharge many patients from state-sponsored mental hospitals into the community. To support the deinstitutionalized mentally ill, the Community Mental Health Act was passed in 1963 and amended in 1965 to provide grants for the initial costs of staffing newly constructed mental health centers to provide care for the mentally ill on an outpatient basis (House 1989).

Communities across the United States, however, were not equipped to house this ill yet ambulatory population. As a result, many of the deinstitutionalized elderly ended up in nursing homes, while many of the younger group were placed in board-and-care facilities (House 1989) or became homeless. Morrissey (1982) maintains that the deinstitutionalization movement has had a major impact on the proliferation of board-and-care homes. Today, many of the younger patients who moved from mental institutions to board-and-care homes are aging in place.

Only since 1940 has board-and-care been linked with care for the elderly, following the enactment of the Social Security Act in 1935. The Social Security Program (SSP) enabled older persons to purchase board-and-care services and marked the creation of public responsibility for the dependent in American society (Capitman 1989). One of the first references in the literature to the aged in foster care homes was by Aptekar (1965), who mentioned it as a comparatively recent development (McCoin 1983).

Issues Facing Contemporary Board-and-Care Homes

Financing Board-and-Care Services

Board-and-care homes are financed both with private funds, on a fee-for-service basis, and with public monies, for those who cannot afford to purchase services on their own. The public funding and the risk of expanding public costs have remained the source of most concern to policymakers.

Social Security and SSI (the federally mandated income-maintenance program) provide the financial basis for dependent adults with limited economic resources to purchase board-and-care services (Capitman 1989). These payments are made to the individual elder (or a representative payee) as income that is then used to pay for care, instead of reimbursing the facility for services rendered, as is done in nursing homes. Capitman (1989) noted that financing board-and-care services through income support to beneficiaries, rather than vendor payments to facilities for services rendered, has had several consequences.

First, no information is readily available on either the characteristics of SSI/SSP recipients in board-and-care facilities or patterns of public investment in this type of care. Second, there is no mechanism to reimburse facilities for targeting services to client need or to influence the quality and efficiency of care delivered. These consequences have, in turn, resulted in wide variations in definitions and programs from state to state. In California, for example, board-and-care homes developed ad hoc, yet served 82 percent of the state's sheltered care population and comprised 72 percent of the state's facilities. This led Segal and Aviram (1978) to conclude that board-and-care homes represented a new residential care system for the mentally ill in California.

In addition, Medicaid plays a role in financing board-and-care services (Capitman 1989). SSI recipients are categorically eligible for Medicaid, although states have some ability to vary coverage. Some states cover board-and-care services through traditional Medicaid programs such as personal care provider programs, and some supplement board-and-care through reimbursement of adult day care. Moreover, some facilities that are licensed for both nursing home care, which is reimbursable, and lower levels of care, which are not reimbursable, shift some costs between levels of care. In these situations, Medicaid may indirectly cover some board-and-care costs.

Several states (e.g., Washington, Wisconsin, Colorado, and Oregon) use Medicaid 2176 Home- and Community-Based Services Waivers to cover some of the costs of board-and-care. Oregon, for example, uses this method to pay for adult foster care services for older adults "who are financially eligible and technically eligible for nursing care based on their functional needs" (Kane and Kane 1988, 3–4).

Capitman (1989) suggests several strengths and weaknesses in using Medicaid funds to pay for board-and-care services. This approach to funding may result in better-coordinated health and social services by integrating board-and-care into the medically oriented long-term care system. However, this approach does not guarantee cost containment and may diminish the homelike atmosphere of these facilities.

Regulating Board-and-Care Homes

Board-and-care regulation falls under conflicting and overlapping local, state, and national jurisdictions. At the federal level, regulatory policy addressing the board-and-care industry has been limited and largely ineffective (Lyon 1993). The Keys amendment, passed by Congress in 1976, requires states to establish, maintain, and enforce standards in institutions or other group-living arrangements in which a significant number of SSI recipients reside or are likely to reside. This legislation has been largely ineffective in assuring standardization in such facilities (Baggett 1989). The only enforcement mechanism built into the Keys amendment is the reduction of the SSI payment to the resident of a facility that does not meet state standards. This provision punishes the resident for noncompliance on the part of the provider (Reichstein and Bergofsky 1983). Consequently, states have been reluctant to report abuses, thus undermining the effectiveness of the act (Conley 1989; Reichstein and Bergofsky 1980).

In a nationwide study using 1980 data, Mor, Sherwood, and Gutkin (1986) described the regulatory status of residential care homes. The large institutions in their study were generally regulated by state health departments, while smaller homes were regulated, if at all, by a mix of programs administered by various state agencies (e.g., aging, disabilities, housing, health care, income maintenance, and adult protection) (Dobkin 1989; Mor, Sherwood, and Gutkin 1986; Reichstein and Bergofsky 1983; Sherman and Newman 1988). In Maryland, residential care programs for up to fifteen persons are regulated by separate state agencies for health, human resources, and aging, as well as by some individual jurisdictions within the state (Dobkin 1989). Each agency sets it own requirements for the minimum size for regulatory oversight, ranging from one to twenty-one residents, with the most frequent minimum being one or three (GAO 1989).

The confusion regarding board-and-care homes, especially the smaller homes, results from their marginal status between the jurisdictions of several agencies and bureaucracies (Morgan, Eckert, and Lyon 1993). Since these homes house different types of dependent populations, various state and local agencies become involved in monitoring, certifying, or regulating them. Thus, the responsibility rests with everyone and no one (Baggett 1989).

Comparing Board-and-Care with Other Long-Term Care Options

The small board-and-care home represents one alternative currently filling the gap between home and nursing home for dependent adults who require assistance in activities of daily living but do not require skilled nursing care. They differ from institutional settings (i.e., nursing homes) in that "their primary purpose is to provide nonmedical personal care" (McCoy and Conley 1990, 148). Thus, board-and-care homes serve a less-impaired population that requires supervision and support in activities of daily living (see chap. 5). Board-and-care homes are also generally smaller than nursing homes, with the largest approaching the sizes of nursing homes, but the bulk of homes found to be much smaller (Dobkin 1989; Hawes et al. 1993). The cost of care is generally considerably lower than that in nursing homes, an issue especially important to individuals with few financial resources who are ineligible for Medicaid support (Chen 1989; Ehrlich 1986). Although many board-and-care homes are privately operated, as are nursing homes, profit in many of the smaller homes is minimal at best (Chen 1989; Habenstein, Kiefer, and Wang 1976). The environments within these small homes are more personalized, may provide a greater chance for autonomy, and are less regulated and regimented by rules than are typical nursing homes (Diamond 1992; Rubinstein 1995; Savishinsky 1991). As care settings, then, small board-and-care homes represent a sharp contrast with the well-understood environment of the nursing home.

Care in board-and-care homes also differs from independent living (i.e., in one's own home and/or with kin) in that the homes provide some degree of personal oversight for people who would otherwise forgo this service if living alone (Rubinstein 1995). As reported in a study of board-and-care homes conducted in Missouri, families considered them a more desirable living arrangement than nursing homes when frail or impaired persons were unable to care for themselves or when relatives could not provide care (Habenstein, Kiefer, and Wang 1976).

Board-and-care is also currently compared with the new phenomenon known as assisted living. Assisted living housing can be defined as a model of residential long-term care based on the concept of outfitting a residential environment with professionally delivered personal care services in a way that avoids institutionalization and keeps older frail individuals independent as long as possible (Regnier, Hamilton, and Yatabe 1991).

As a housing type between congregate housing and skilled nursing care, it serves the needs of persons with less severe mental and physical problems.

As noted by Rubinstein (1995), confusion in terminology exists among assisted living, board-and-care, and personal care or supervised care homes (Health Care Investments Analysts 1992). The label *assisted living* has been used to differentiate this type of housing from conventional board-and-care housing (Kane, Wilson, and Clemmer 1993). The term carries none of the baggage of past problems or the negative connotations that board-and-care has accumulated in the minds of many (see Kane, Wilson, and Clemmer 1993; Regnier, Hamilton, and Yatabe 1991). In fact, Kane, Wilson, and Clemmer (1993), in describing board-and-care homes, dismiss them as uniformly of poor quality, contrasting them with newer (and presumably higher-quality) assisted living settings. While board-and-care homes tend to be small and informal community-based settings, assisted living facilities tend to be larger, ranging from twenty-five to over one hundred persons (Golant 1992). Small board-and-care homes are family-style arrangements in which residents usually coreside with their caregivers. Such small homes often operate without professional management assistance (Regnier, Hamilton, and Yatabe 1991).

The primary difference between these two types of housing/care options is related to the physical environment. Ideally, assisted living settings have private living quarters, such as efficiency apartments, with doors that can be locked for privacy. The small board-and-care homes, in contrast, while often offering private rooms, do not have doors that can be locked or separate kitchens and bathing facilities.

This fundamental environmental difference is important, since it is directly related to the costs of operation (Chen 1989). The high start-up costs involved in a purpose-built or purpose-modified facility mean that residents in assisted living facilities would, undoubtedly, be paying higher fees than many of the residents in small board-and-care homes (Chen 1989). In fact, research has shown this to be the case for current assisted living facilities, where the range of fees is considerably higher than those we found in the small board-and-care homes (Kane, Wilson, and Clemmer 1993).

Social Marginality

The concept of social marginality emerged as a useful way to make sense of the findings on the small homes we studied in Cleveland and Baltimore. The small board-and-care home reflects aspects of social marginality in terms of being caught between the housing and health care systems (Baggett 1989); operator/resident relationships are neither traditional family bonds nor typical professional/client bonds, and the residents are marked as marginal to the dominant group by their lack of strong ties to the social order (Dobkin 1989). This marginality, in turn, may have serious implications for individuals within the homes and for the board-and-care homes in the larger societal context of neighborhoods and regulatory and funding agencies (Morgan, Eckert, and Lyon 1993).

As we will show, both the operators and residents of small board-and-care homes are victims of, and sometimes benefit from, marginality. In the case of the residents, experiences with mental illness, poverty, and truncated family systems contribute to weak linkages with the dominant institutions of society; making them "outsiders" (Birkel and Jones 1989; Soldo 1981).

Residents are also marginalized between the healthy and the ill. Most residents have chronic physical and/or mental conditions that prohibit their independent living without substantial support. Thus, they are not "healthy" in the functional sense, nor are they "ill" in the medical sense. Their conditions, for the most part, do not require regular medical intervention, and the care that they require is mostly supervisory and personal, that is, assistance with the tasks of everyday living. Society recognizes a responsibility to treat the ill, providing interventions such as Medicaid to assist those individuals too poor to get necessary medical attention, but expects the healthy to be independent. Residents of small board-and-care homes fall between the cracks by virtue of not being sufficiently ill, physically or mentally, to clearly warrant such societal support.

Although sometimes argued to be powerful relative to their residents, the operators of small board-and-care homes are often marginal to the dominant groups of society as well. Some of them mirror the disadvantages of those in their care, such as having little education, spotty work histories, and limited family support systems (i.e., divorced or widowed). Moreover, their work as providers, unaffiliated with formal systems of care, places them outside the mainstream of paraprofessional work in health care.

Operators and the homes themselves are marginal in that they exist between family and professional providers, with the rights of neither group, but with the duties of both with regard to their residents. As we will see in chapter 4, operators report being caught in conflicts between regulators and residents or between residents and their families.

In their communities, homes are subject to zoning hearings and community pressures, since they are marginal to their communities as nonfamilial residences. In some cases, neighborhoods have the right to force the operator to cease board-and-care work or to relocate to a neighborhood where such "commercial" activities are permitted. By fitting into the mold of neither single-family residences nor businesses, small board-and-care homes are subject to pressures of marginality that may threaten their continued existence.

We argue that the homes, their operators and residents, and their interactions with the larger society are shaped in a very real sense by social marginality—being between the worlds of family and nursing home, healthy and ill, residential and service environments. The marginal status of small board-and-care homes may have certain positive consequences in that their invisibility may have enabled them to develop in a grass-roots fashion (Morgan, Eckert, and Lyon 1993). By having no clear agency with a mandate over small board-and-care homes, regulators have overlooked them through much of their history. This limited regulatory oversight has allowed more varied, personalized services and environments to evolve than might have been the case under strict rules and regulations (see Appelbaum and Ritchie 1992; Habenstein, Kiefer, and Wang 1976; Segal and Hwang 1994 for the negative effects of regulation on small board-and-care homes in three states).

Insider and Outsider Perspectives

Many of the problems and contrasting points of view surrounding the board-and-care industry result, in part, from its marginal status. Small board-and-care homes are judged by two seemingly incompatible sets of criteria: their medical/human services qualities and their "homelike" qualities (Rubinstein 1995). By virtue of their roles and responsibilities, health and human services professionals, policymakers, and program administrators are primarily concerned with the formal, bureaucratic aspects of board-and-care homes (safety, public and private financing, and the medical and social services aspects of these settings), while operators and residents emphasize the domestic, primary group, and familial nature of the homes. Given these competing criteria, one way to approach the multiple definitions of small board-and-care homes is to contrast the perspectives and concerns of those who work and live outside these settings (the outsider's perspective) with those who operate and reside in them (the insider's perspective).

The dominant cultural view of board-and-care homes is shaped by persons external to the environment: health and human services professionals, policymakers, program administrators, and the media.

Health and human services personnel, such as case managers, nurses, and social workers, view board-and-care from a clinical perspective arising from their professional training. Their socially sanctioned role is to assess the individual's needs for services and the ability of various providers within the formal system of human services to meet those needs.

The characteristics of small board-and-care homes separate them from the types of facilities formally approved by the professional service system. Their care is more akin to that provided in the domestic domains of family and friends than to the care in formal organizations such as nursing homes. Although demonstrating many primary group characteristics, small board-and-care homes are not treated as families when they are encountered by the professional service sector. Instead, they are viewed as mini–nursing homes. As such, the issues and concerns raised by health and human services professionals who work with operators and residents of board-and-care homes include the training and competence of operators, the adequacy and quality of the physical environment and services, and the appropriateness of placement. Measured by formal bureaucratic standards, many small board-and-care homes are perceived as substandard living and care environments.

Policymakers and program administrators respond, in large measure, to negative publicity and the abuses believed to be widespread among small board-and-care homes. Their historically and socially sanctioned response is to rationalize the care delivery system through the development and implementation of regulations (see Estes 1979).

Major issues for policymakers and program administrators include how to supply high-quality board-and-care housing through the development of programs, monitoring, and regulatory oversight. They are also concerned with how to finance the custodial care of dependent adults, reimburse to maximize fiscal oversight while maintaining quality care and autonomy for residents, coordinate financing among diverse funding sources, and save money. Policy concerns involving the operators focus on how to weed out or avoid those who perform poorly. Policymakers and program administrators are also concerned with the well-being and rights of residents.

In light of the issues confronting these groups, it is not surprising that much of the research on board-and-care to date has focused on regulation and reimbursement in multistate, national, or single-state studies (Reichstein and Bergofsky 1983; Dittmar et al. 1983; Hawes et al. 1993).

These studies are limited, however, by the lack of information about those homes *not* under some regulatory or licensing authority, often housing smaller numbers of residents. None of these studies provide information on the realities of small board-and-care homes from the perspectives of operators and residents. This fact has led McCoy and Conley (1990),

Eckert and Lyon (1992), and others to point out that our current conceptual and research frameworks for examining housing and supportive services to the frail elderly do not adequately include small board-and-care homes.

The public's perception of small board-and-care homes is largely dependent upon what people read, hear, or see in the popular media. The Select Committee on Aging, U.S. House of Representatives report "Board and Care Homes in America: A National Tragedy" references over seventy newspaper articles on various aspects of life in board-and-care homes (1989). While several of these articles allude to well-run, high-quality homes, they soon turn to the seamy side of board-and-care life. For example, board-and-care homes were typically described as "deadly," "cockroach heavens," "asylums," and "dumping grounds" (House 1989). The report concluded that

> the Nation's over 1 million elderly, disabled, and mentally ill currently residing in board and care homes in America are frequently the victims of fraud, neglect and abuse. Warehoused and drugged, this vulnerable population is usually unaware that their rights to board, care and protection can easily be circumscribed by unscrupulous home owners or greedy and uncaring home managers." (Senate 1989, 11).

These sweeping conclusions were based on media coverage of board-and-care homes, surveys of ombudsmen whose job it is to respond to cases of abuse and neglect, and subcommittee staff visits (accompanied by regulatory officials) to selected homes in nine states and the District of Columbia. After reading the report, one is struck by the negative bias toward all forms of board-and-care services that fall outside traditional regulatory structures. No scientific rigor was used to select homes for visits and examination. Yet, the visual and verbal profiles of the forty-six licensed and unlicensed homes visited conveyed only one image, that of a "nationwide board and care problem of baffling proportions" (House 1989, 82).

As a result of the overly negative bias in media reports on board-and-care housing, public concerns include how to ensure a safe and protective environment, ensure that public dollars are well spent, avoid the fraud documented in some board-and-care homes, finance board-and-care as a community-based residential care option, and protect residents from poor-quality operators.

Limited Knowledge of Insiders' Views

Very few studies examine the insiders' world of board-and-care homes on the microlevel, from an interactionist perspective. This viewpoint takes the orientation of those most intimately involved in board-and-care housing:

the operators and the residents. In examining whether foster care homes are "family" homes or mini-institutions, Sherman and Newman (1988) suggested that the foster care families they studied could be termed surrogate families, on the basis of operators' perceptions of the interpersonal relationships in the homes.

Studies of small board-and-care homes (Eckert, Namazi, and Kahana 1987; Sherman and Newman 1988) have found them to be much like typical family settings in single-family homes. The majority of operators were middle-aged women, many of whom had limited education, as is characteristic of women providing direct care to dependent adults in other settings (Abel and Nelson 1990). In addition to clients, most operators had other family members living with them in their homes, adding to a familial atmosphere.

As further elaborated in chapters 2 and 6, the *operators* characterized their homes as familylike environments in which they shared activities and affection with residents as well as giving one-on-one care (Sherman and Newman 1988; Morgan, Eckert, and Lyon 1993). A common theme in the few studies of the interaction within small board-and-care homes is that caregivers are motivated to provide care by humanitarian aims, strong religious convictions, and a wish to keep elderly residents out of nursing homes (Oktay and Volland 1981; Mor, Sherwood, and Gutkin 1986; Sherman and Newman 1988). Very few operators are reported to think of their homes as a business, even though certain business aspects necessarily intrude. From the perspective of operators, what they do does not fit with the more institutional definitions of housing and care espoused by outsiders.

The issues of concern to operators reflect their multiple roles as direct caregivers, bridges between residents' families and health/human service professionals, and managers of small businesses. Operators' concerns for the board-and-care environment include how to maintain and improve the physical environment for residents, meet various regulatory requirements on limited funds, avoid negative reactions from the local community, and locate appropriate clients. Financial issues confronting the board-and-care home operators focus on ensuring sufficient financial return to continue operation, meeting the financial needs of residents (e.g., health care, personal spending, clothing needs), and maximizing the regularity and reliability of payment. Finally, operators must concern themselves with how to determine their limits for providing care to increasingly frail or ill residents, manage personal attachments to residents, and remove problematic residents from the home.

Studies from the perspective of *residents or clients* of small board-and-care homes are rare. Previous analyses of the data reported here give an initial clue about how residents perceive their homes and situations (Eckert, Lyon, and Namazi 1990). In an examination of how older individuals make themselves feel at home in small board-and-care environments, residents reported that the opportunity for exchange of affection and an atmosphere of sharing, responsibility, and interaction were very important in their definitions of the board-and-care environment as a home (Namazi et al. 1991). The relationship between the operator and resident was found to be important in how positively the resident perceived the home environment as well as feelings of personal well-being (Namazi et al. 1989).

Based on our current understanding, the issues confronting residents of board-and-care include how to locate affordable care appropriate to their level of functioning and how to maximize autonomy and privacy in that environment. Maximizing their rights in an imbalanced power relationship and maintaining control of finances (when appropriate) within the board-and-care environment are other key issues for residents. Finally, residents are faced with the challenge of fostering amicable relationships with coresidents in the home.

The Research Process

While there is an extensive literature characterizing the physical and social context of formal long-term care institutions, such as nursing homes and homes for the aged (Lawton 1980; Johnson and Grant 1985), previous research has not focused on the physical and social milieu of the small board-and-care home and the psychosocial well-being of residents. At the time our research program began, very little was known of the microenvironment of small board-and-care homes (McCoin 1983; Sherman and Newman 1977; Streib, Folts, and Hilker 1984). To address the gap in our understanding of these small homes, a program of research was begun in Cleveland, Ohio, in 1983 and continued in Baltimore, Maryland, into the early 1990s.

The research design and approach to studying small board-and-care homes was modeled after that of an earlier eight-year longitudinal study of older, single-room occupancy (SRO) hotel dwellers (Eckert 1980). Eckert characterized this elsewhere as an "ethnographic research process," in which the procedures used and questions asked become increasingly focused through time (Eckert 1987). Figure 1 is a visual representation of the process. In the beginning stages, research, exploration, detailed description, and understanding of the social organization of the setting are of prime concern. Initial information serves as the basis for design of subsequent research questions and methodologies for addressing them. As the

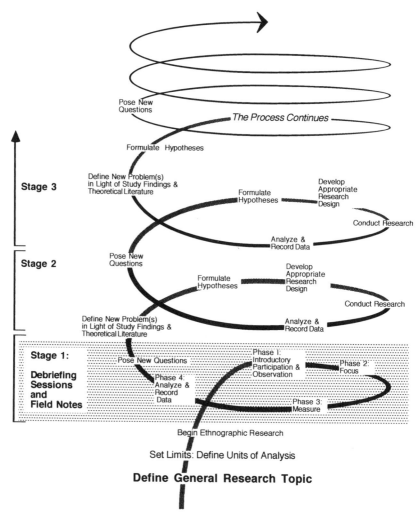

Fig. 1. Ethnographic Research Process
Source: Reinharz and Rowles, 1988, p. 243.

research process unfolds, greater emphasis is placed on explanation through the testing of hypotheses related to relevant theoretical constructs and questions. Thus, the process moves from general to specific questions and inductive to deductive methodologies over time, with the accumulation of pertinent information. The research on small board-and-care homes involved both qualitative and quantitative methodologies aimed at detailed description and explanation.

One problem with early studies involving board-and-care was that they lumped together facilities that varied in size, services rendered, populations served, and the levels of care required by residents. Based on pilot research conducted in Ohio, the smaller homes (e.g., three to twenty-five residents), expected to offer a therapeutic, homelike atmosphere (Blake 1987; Donahue and Oriol 1981), were judged to deserve special attention. Despite definitional complexities, these small homes were believed to share common characteristics.

The data presented in subsequent chapters derive from two related research studies of small board-and-care homes, conducted between 1983 and 1992 in Cleveland, Ohio, and Baltimore, Maryland. In each case, the metropolitan areas (i.e., cities and their surrounding counties) provided the frame for locating and selecting homes for participation in the research projects. Both are midsized cities in the eastern half of the country, and we do not contend that they are representative of small board-and-care homes nationally. The level of detail on the insider's perspective on these small homes is, nonetheless, unmatched in existing research. (For a more detailed discussion of research methodology, see the appendix.)

The Cleveland Study

The purpose of the initial study was to learn much more about the life inside small board-and-care homes. Key research goals included describing the homes from the perspectives of operators and residents; profiling the physical and social environments of the homes and determining how these affected older residents' psychosocial well-being and satisfaction; and discovering the links between the health and demographics of residents, their satisfaction with the home, and their psychological well-being.

Since the homes were legally unlicensed (Ohio had no regulations governing small homes at that time) (Hawes et al. 1993), they were difficult to locate and recruit for participation (see the appendix). Many of the homes that were found did not meet the criterion of housing fewer than twenty-five residents, at least one of whom was aged sixty or older. The age criterion was later lowered to forty-five, adding a few additional homes.

Data were collected from both operators and residents in structured, focused interviews conducted by experienced and trained interviewers. Questions to operators addressed the physical character of the home, acceptability of various types of residents, rules in the home, types of records kept, social interaction in the homes, services offered, and their motivations for operating a home. Resident interviews paralleled operator interviews in addressing physical and social aspects of the living environment, but added social supports, the homelike and familylike aspects of the home, recent losses, physical and mental health, psychological well-being, and environmental satisfaction. Many residents could not be interviewed because of a variety of problems and limitations, reducing the generalizability of their responses (see chap. 5).

This book offers the most in-depth analysis on numerous issues drawn from the Cleveland study, and the data from Cleveland operators and residents will be apparent throughout the chapters to follow. Limitations in this initial study focused attention on modifying the methodological approach in the second study, which was subsequently undertaken in Baltimore.

The Baltimore Study

In 1987 the study of small board-and-care homes was expanded to Baltimore. Again the sample focused on small, legally unlicensed homes. The focus in the second study was on the operators and how they managed the constant care of multiply impaired individuals. Our major initial hypotheses concerned burden and burnout among the operators of small board-and-care homes.

To gain a more in-depth understanding of the environment in these homes, to follow up on issues raised by the findings in Cleveland, and to fill gaps in knowledge from the study there, a different methodology was developed. The change involved using a longitudinal design of repeated interviews (four at six-month intervals) with the operators ($N = 103$). In addition, health evaluations were conducted on selected older residents. This strategy both provided detailed information on health status unavailable from the question-and-answer format of an interview and permitted more-impaired persons to participate, giving a more realistic view of the range of health conditions among the residents than was available in the Cleveland study.

Health evaluations of eighty-five older residents were completed by nurses with graduate gerontological training. Operators and others assisted those who were cognitively impaired or otherwise unable to communicate. Many of the items, however, were observations (e.g., vital signs, use of hearing aid, walker, or other assistive devices). Questions on activities of daily living and other functional status items were bolstered by a medication profile and a checklist of major symptoms.

Aside from the issue of operator burden, the repeated interviews with the operators each had different themes and ranged from forty to ninety minutes (on average) in duration. The first interview focused on the operator's background and motivation, formal and informal supports, and resident information. Financial issues and physical aspects of the environment were at the core of the second interview, while the third addressed social interactions, departures, and orientations toward altruism. The fourth and final interview emphasized regulation and regulators, rules within the home, quality of the environment, respite, and community acceptance. In each interview we also gathered limited information about residents ($N = 342$), including some new arrivals to the homes during the study.

All of these interviews, as well as the health evaluations of the older (aged sixty or above) residents, were conducted inside the homes, giving the interviewers the opportunity to observe the ongoing routine and interactions among those residing there. In addition, the repeated visits by the same interviewer developed rapport, which proved invaluable in getting detailed and honest answers to some very difficult questions. The repeated interviews also enabled use of the early data in developing themes and issues for subsequent visits, enriching the data collection.

Repeated interviewing in a longitudinal study also creates the opportunity for attrition. Initially, 103 home operators who met our criteria of having eight or fewer residents and coresiding in the home were interviewed. We maintained 87 percent of these operators as participants through the eighteen-month interviewing period, losing the most between the first and second interviews.

Project HOME

To bolster an unexpectedly meager sampling frame in Baltimore, small homes from a state-run program (Project HOME/CARE, hereafter referred to as Project HOME) were added to the sample. These regulated homes closely resembled the nonregulated homes already in the sample, but they differed in some important ways. Project HOME involves an integrated model of regulation (Mor, Sherwood, and Gutkin 1986), monitoring quality while providing support to home operators and residents. Central to the program is the SSI supplementation given to its participating residents, who were originally restricted to deinstitutionalized mentally ill persons. The program was expanded to include all types of disabled adults and now has 35 percent of its participants over age sixty-five. In the early 1990s, the program still served a population consisting primarily of chronically mentally ill individuals, a younger and more male population than is found in the remainder of the board-and-care industry. Homes participating in this program are restricted to three residents, operators receive training, and residents have case managers overseeing their services in the homes and other programs (day-care, job training, etc.) in which they participate. During the time we were collecting data, the subsidies to SSI from Project HOME were the highest in the country, making a substantial difference to the economic well-being of the home (Dobkin 1989). Because of these important differences, homes and residents participating in Project HOME are often differentiated in the analyses that follow.

In the chapters that follow, analysis moves between the Cleveland and Baltimore data. Sometimes, comparisons are made between the board-and-care homes, the operators, and the residents in Cleveland and Baltimore, and at other times, only data from a single location are available on a select topic. As a result of the greater amount of data collected with the longitudinal research design, the Baltimore study was the major source of data for most of the analyses.

Seeing Board-and-Care through Different Lenses

The lenses through which one views board-and-care sharply delineate the aspects of the environment that come into focus and the issues and concerns that come to be defined as salient. Those who view board-and-care from the outside see it as a care setting that needs to be integrated into the formal long-term care network and the professional service system. As currently conceived, this system is organized on a medical model of care. This model is typified by the formal role of the physician, who occupies the top of the hierarchy in nursing homes as well as in home care. Even though physicians have little direct contact with patients in most nursing home and home care settings, their decisions are legally binding (Johnson and Grant 1985). From the perspective of many professionals, program administrators, and policymakers, board-and-care homes are "bootleg nursing homes." Thus, in their view, rationalization and formalization of board-and-care services through existing models and policies wi'l address issues of quality assurance, the nature of the services provided, financing, supply, and protection of the residents' rights.

By contrast, both the operators and the residents appear to emphasize board-and-care as a home or place of residence. They discuss the social relationships and caregiving aspects of day-to-day life in the home. From their viewpoint, caring is enmeshed in the domestic domain of family and friends, rather than in the formal relationships and arrangements typical of organizations such as nursing homes.

Our focus, then, was on the microenvironment of small board-and-care homes, and most especially on the operators. As the "linchpins" in these settings (Newman 1989), they were the major sources of information for constructing the reality of board-and-care homes. Through their eyes we can begin to understand the challenges facing board-and-care as a marginal industry between the family and the nursing home.

The issues and concerns associated with the position of board-and-care

2 □ The Board-and-Care Environment

□ The physical environment of small board-and-care homes is unfamiliar to most of us, although there may be such homes operating anonymously in our own communities. In this chapter we focus on physical and spatial aspects of the small homes that house a small number of persons each but may constitute up to two-thirds of board-and-care homes nationally (Sherwood, Morris, and Sherwood 1986; Newcomer and Grant 1988). The opportunities and constraints built into the physical and service environment demonstrate the homes' marginality by the way they straddle the boundaries between traditional family life and the more institutional environments in which most long-term care is provided. This marginality between family and formal organization is often apparent in the physical environment and use of space in the homes.

The quality of the home, including its physical environment and services, is the topic of considerable public policy debate. The desire to enhance quality and protect residents from harm is generally the impetus for the development of both regulatory policies and funding programs. But consensus about how to evaluate quality has not been achieved. It is difficult to establish successful outcomes for the clients housed in small board-and-care homes. This lack of standards for desired outcomes is understandable for a resident population characterized by multiple impairments, both physical and mental (Newman 1989; Reschovsky and Ruchlin 1993). When maintaining current levels of function or minimizing anticipated decline in residents with chronic and degenerative conditions (e.g., Alzheimer's disease) are the goals of long-term care, measurement of outcomes is problematic at best. Many of the intangible, but valued, elements of high-quality social interaction (e.g., availability of the staff to residents or familial qualities of the interactions) are also difficult to quantify. Research by Reschovsky and Ruchlin (1993) using 1983 data and a previous analysis from our Baltimore study (Lyon 1993) suggest that there are elements that can be assessed indirectly to measure quality in board-and-care homes. These evaluations focus on structural and process features of the environment, including space and privacy, the physical environment, and fire and other safety provisions (Reschovsky and Ruchlin 1993). Selective aspects of quality have been related to facility size, fee levels, nonprofit in the middle ground between home care and institutional care serve to structure the discussion that follows. Dimensions of the board-and-care home environment comprising physical and household characteristics as well as the issues of control, privacy, autonomy, services, quality, and community acceptance are addressed in chapter 2. Chapter 3 looks at the economics of small board-and-care homes. Topics include the income, expenses, and profitability of providing board-and-care services; operators' attitudes about the financial aspects of their work; and how operators manage money to make ends meet. In chapters 4 and 5, respectively, the characteristics and perspectives of the operators and residents are described and discussed. Chapter 4 addresses several questions. Who are the operators? What are the stresses and burdens associated with providing board-and-care services? What are the rewards of providing care? In chapter 5, we describe the social, physical, and mental status of board-and-care home residents. The social supports available to the operators of small board-and-care homes and the social relationships and interactions within homes are the topic of chapter 6. Chapter 7 concludes with a summary of the key findings and a discussion of the social and political factors that will influence the future of board-and-care services in long-term care.

status, and other traits, but findings are very mixed (e.g., in Reschovsky and Ruchlin [1993], greater staffing levels were associated with *lower*-quality interaction within the home).

Moon (1989, viii) suggests that board-and-care fills in "for the deficiencies of housing for older Americans in an era in which private residences are not well adapted to the needs of the frail or the handicapped and public, medical facilities are increasingly limited to sicker and sicker populations." As a stopgap, policymakers and program administrators try to design strategies that will ensure maximum safety (i.e., minimize risks) for those being cared for in such homes (Hawes et al. 1993). Existing policies pertaining to board-and-care homes in many jurisdictions focus on such issues as fire safety and space requirements, reflecting this interest in minimizing risk (Conley 1989; Feder et al. 1989; Kane, Wilson, and Clemmer 1993; Reichstein and Bergofsky 1983). But the physical environment is more than just a safety issue for the operators and the residents living in small board-and-care homes. As we shall see, the physical context of care reflects the fundamental difference between these homes and the larger, more formally organized institutions currently providing care to dependent adults.

The purpose of this chapter is to describe the physical features of the homes, the composition of the households, the services that are provided, and some aspects of everyday life that pertain to the physical environment. These features describe the context in which care is provided and in which relationships are developed in the homes (see also chap. 6). Viewing the context of the care, the physical environment, and its social structure in which the interaction between home operator and resident occurs, reinforces the social marginality of small board-and-care homes in a variety of ways.

The Physical Environment in Small Homes

Even given the restriction on home size in our samples (as described in chapter 1—homes had between one and eight residents), most of the board-and-care homes we studied in both cities were at the lower end (one to three residents) of these size ranges. Although all of our homes could be described as small, as we will see, size makes a difference, even among the "small." Over one-fifth of Baltimore homes (21.4 percent) had only one resident, another 31.1 percent reported two residents at the first interview, and one-third (33.0 percent) had three, for a total of 85.4 percent of Baltimore homes having three or fewer residents. In Cleveland the distribution was somewhat broader, with almost one-quarter (24.5 percent) of homes having one resident, one in five (20.9 percent) reporting two, and slightly fewer (18.7 percent, 14.4 percent, and 12.9 percent, respectively) reporting three, four, or five residents in their homes at the time of the interview. In all, 78.4 percent of Cleveland homes housed four or fewer dependent adults. This places most of the homes we studied at the "mom-and-pop" end of the size continuum, in contrast to the larger homes studied in most of the prior research (see Dittmar et al. 1983; Mor, Sherwood, and Gutkin 1986).

In addition, this small size exempted most of the homes from regulation, which also differentiates these homes from those in most prior studies (see Newman and Thompson 1987). The most closely comparable sample of homes is from the work of Sherman and Newman (1988), who studied adult foster care homes of similar sizes and environmental characteristics, albeit serving somewhat different resident populations (i.e., homes designated for mentally retarded, mentally ill, and elderly) and clearly regulated by the state. The work of Sherman and Newman provides the most direct comparison with the physical environments we are describing in Cleveland and Baltimore.

Homes in both of our samples often had vacancies. Only 19.4 percent of Cleveland homes, contrasted with 43.7 percent of Baltimore homes, were full or slightly beyond their capacities (by one or two residents) when the operators were initially interviewed. Most of the operators reported relatively few vacancies (47.6 percent in Baltimore had one or two slots, while about 73.3 percent of Cleveland homes had four or fewer vacancies) at that first interview. This modest vacancy rate is bounded, of course, by the small overall size of the homes we studied. Strategies for and attitudes about filling these vacancies are discussed further in chapter 4.

According to open-ended responses to questions asked of the Baltimore operators, determination of the maximum number of residents in their homes was primarily a function of regulation (mentioned by 58.3 percent of operators) and the physical size of and number of rooms in the house (mentioned by 41.7 percent of operators). Many operators said that they felt capable of caring for more clients but were constrained by regulations and physical size limits (e.g., number of bedrooms, bathrooms) from housing more residents than they currently did. For instance, one exemplary operator in Baltimore would have been able to care for more people in her home by utilizing third-floor bedrooms, but she could not afford to install a required fire escape to permit residents to be housed on that floor. Only 13.6 percent of home operators mentioned the care demands of residents as important in determining how many they could accept.

The types of housing stock chosen for providing board-and-care is, for the most part, typical of residential communities. In Cleveland most were single-family homes (75.5 percent) or duplexes (15.8 percent) located in a variety of neighborhoods from inner-city urban to suburban and rural, as has been the case in prior research on larger homes (Dittmar et al. 1983; Mor, Sherwood, and Gutkin 1986). The relative absence of larger structures, such as converted apartment buildings, reflects the small-scale operations that have been our research focus. Although, as discussed below, the housing had sometimes been modified to accommodate care of residents, these modifications are often not apparent from the street. Most of the homes easily blend in with those in the surrounding community and do not seem "institutional" or different in any visible way.

In fact, many of the homes are the same ones that the operators have occupied for years while raising their families. In Baltimore, 87.9 percent of operators were owners or were buying their homes, with nearly three-quarters (73.3 percent) still paying on a mortgage. Among home owners, the great majority (79.1 percent) were already living in their current houses when they began providing board-and-care services. Correspondingly, few Baltimore operators (12.1 percent) reported that they had acquired the house to start offering board-and-care services. This contrasts rather strikingly with the notion of purpose-built (or purpose-modified) housing facilities common in more institutional types of long-term care. It also contrasts with the emerging concept of assisted living, where definitions often turn on having purpose-built facilities (Mollica et al. 1992). In many cases, these board-and-care homes were simply converted from other uses, often raising the operator's own children, to care for dependent adults and elders.

In many cases, however, the operators had made some changes in the physical aspects of their homes to enhance their ability to provide care or to gain additional space. When we asked Baltimore operators about modifications to their homes, over half (60.2 percent) reported making such changes. The most common home changes or improvements that were made in connection with caregiving were modifications to or the addition of a bathroom (19.4 percent) and the addition of space or rooms to the home (12.7 percent)(see fig. 2). There were a few differences across types of homes, with white operators more likely than their African American counterparts to have made improvements in a kitchen, and larger homes (13.3 percent) much more likely than the smallest homes (0 percent) to have added bathrooms. Most of these modifications were done by contractors, with costs ranging from $0 to $40,000, but averaging around $2,000 (median in 1990 dollars).

Operators often demonstrated pride in the physical environments they provided, including "showing off" renovations to our interviewers. As one interviewer reports, "The operator took me on another tour of the

Percentage of homes

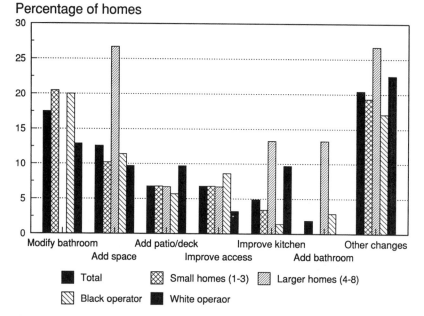

Fig. 2. Prior Home Modifications in Baltimore by Home Size and Race

home to show me her remodeling efforts. The kitchen was completely redone. A portion of the wall which looks out into the main dining room was glassed in and a portable gate was at the kitchen door to keep clients out. (T)he operator also took me through the sitting room. She is in the process of remodeling it. She has enlarged the area by knocking out a wall to an adjoining bedroom."

Despite the improvements that had been made by many operators, few were completely satisfied with the physical environments of their homes at the time of the interviews in Baltimore. While few (10.1 percent) reported that specific physical features of their houses made care more difficult, many expressed interest in making additional improvements to the physical environment. Figure 3 outlines the changes desired by Baltimore operators. Among the changes that were still desired in their homes, 17.5 percent of operators wanted to add rooms or more space, 14.6 percent wanted to add or change a bathroom, and 9.7 percent desired a single-level floor plan, with a few operators suggesting various other changes. Operators with four or more residents were significantly more likely (13.3 percent vs. 0 percent) to desire to add a deck or patio in the future. Clearly, these operators are mentioning modifications that would be enhancements to already functional environments, rather than basic repairs and fundamen-

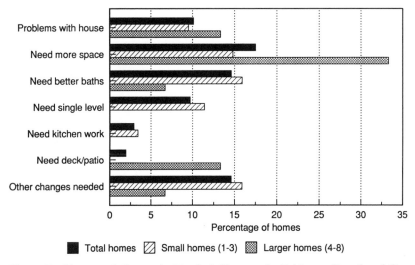

Fig. 3. Problems and Currently Needed Changes in Baltimore Board-and-Care Homes

tal changes to create a minimum standard of living. As later information will show, most of the homes were already in sound physical shape, according to our interviewers.

Composition of the Board-and-Care Household

It is obvious that the operator and residents live in these small residential care homes together, since coresidence was a sample selection criterion. But the question remains as to who else, if anyone, shares the household. Presence of others in small homes has not been widely discussed in previous research on board-and-care but may have important effects on the dynamics of the household. If there are additional members of the household, on the one hand, they may assist in providing services to the dependent adults residing there, share in activities with residents, or simply enhance the sense of a familial environment. Alternatively, coresiding family members or friends may add to the work load of the operator, if she must also provide services (e.g., housekeeping and transportation) for them. Thus, the needs of family members may compete with those of residents for attention and emotional support, or their presence may support the operator in providing necessary care to residents. In addition, the presence of paid staff persons in the homes, whether or not they "live in," influences the provision of services and the dynamics of interaction occurring within the homes.

Coresiding Family Members

Both the first interview with Baltimore home operators and those with Cleveland-area home operators inquired about other individuals residing in the home at that time. The results indicate that there are commonly others (beyond the operator and residents) sharing the household. Figure 4 outlines the comparative findings on the board-and-care households.

In the two operator samples, about four in ten small board-and-care homes included the operator's spouse and/or children. Spouses (mostly husbands) were more common in households of white operators in Baltimore, where two out of three (67.7 percent) had coresiding spouses. This difference, while not statistically significant, was in the same direction for the operators in Cleveland: more white operators (49.5 percent) married and living with their spouses. Children of the operators were not substantially more or less likely to be present in the various types of homes, but

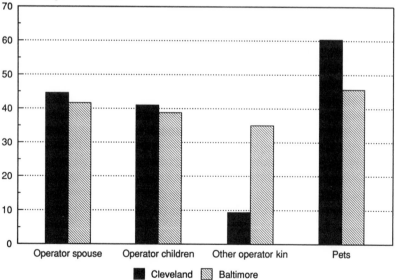

Fig. 4. Household Members Other Than Residents and Operators in Board-and-Care Homes

also were residing in about 40 percent of homes in both cities. Many of the children who were coresiding were not young children; they were more often teens or young adults, who sometimes assisted in the care of the residents. Presence of children cannot, therefore, necessarily be characterized as another burden on the operator's time.

More than one home in three in Baltimore included relatives of the operator other than a spouse or child, and such kin were especially common in larger homes, where they shared in two-thirds (66.7 percent) of the households. Other relatives were less often a part of the household in the Cleveland-area sample (9.4 percent) for reasons that are not clear. Taken together, 70.5 percent of the Cleveland homes studied and a strikingly similar 70.9 percent of the Baltimore homes had at least one person in addition to the operator and the residents in the households. And within these shared households, many (35 percent in Baltimore and 27.3 percent in Cleveland) had two or three types of kin present. White operators were significantly more likely than their African American counterparts to have multiple types of kin in the household. Operators of higher-fee homes in Cleveland were more likely than those in lower-fee homes to have two or more types of kin coresiding in the board-and-care home.

Finally, pets were present in many board-and-care households (see fig. 4). Over 60 percent of the Cleveland homes studied and nearly half of the Baltimore homes included pets of some type. In Baltimore, pets were especially common among the larger homes (71.4 percent) and those operated by whites (67.9 percent), with the significant race difference mirrored also in Cleveland (66.0 percent of white operators reported pets). Pets became an important part of the social life of some homes, with potential therapeutic benefits reflecting those described in the "pet therapy" literature in nursing homes and in the community (see Boldt 1992; Jenkins 1986; Savishinsky 1992). While many nursing homes now have pets as visitors, the residents of most small board-and-care homes can develop an ongoing relationship with a particular pet or pets that may represent a meaningful linkage for an individual with limited social contacts (see chap. 5).

In many cases, the operators told the interviewers how their kin assisted them in their work. Mrs. J., for example, had a daughter and grandson in her household who assisted in the care, primarily by the daughter doing most of the cooking. In another case, an operator and her son ran homes that were across the street from one another. During the day, when the son went to work, his clients would go to his mother's board-and-care home for supervision. Another daughter also lived in this mother's household, assisting in the care of the residents. Assistance from kin was taken for granted by the operators, many of whom relied on kin for respite and emergency support in case of their own illness or incapacity.

Paid Staff

The issue of staffing in these small homes is a difficult one. In many cases the supports described by operators represented a seamless continuum from unpaid, voluntary, and occasional assistance by kin (either within or outside of the household) to the paid support of formal organizations and professionals, such as physicians and nurses. For this research, it was challenging to draw meaningful lines between helpers who were professional and non- or paraprofessional, paid and unpaid, and from the informal network versus formal providers. Our difficulties in this area arose, in part, from the expectations we held that paid staff persons would not be a major component of the support systems of the operators.

We excluded from our definition of staff those individuals that operators described as relatives, friends, neighbors, or health care professionals. Staff persons also had to be paid for their services and present in the home at least weekly to provide some type of services. Results using this definition of paid staff supported our expectations. Nearly three-quarters (72.8 percent) of Baltimore homes reported no member of their support network meeting our definition, with staff size ranging as high as five persons (in three homes). One-half ($N = 14$) of the operators reporting any staff had only one person who could be described as working for pay at least weekly in some role to assist in care of residents. As might be expected, homes with four to eight residents were significantly more likely to have one or more paid staff persons (53.3 percent in larger homes versus 22.7 percent in smaller homes), but there were no differences based on the average fees paid by residents or the home's participation in the Project HOME program. The race of the operator created a difference that approached statistical significance (24.3 percent of African American operators and 32.3 percent of white operators had at least one staff person) but may be an artifact of the already-noted difference in the numbers of residents cared for by operators in each group.

What did these staff persons do to assist the operators? Rather than relying on job titles, we asked operators to specify the tasks for which they paid these staff persons. Sixteen operators mentioned help with housekeeping, followed by ten who had help with "various tasks." Fewer still had help bathing and dressing their residents ($N = 9$), respite care or backup caregiving services ($N = 8$), or assistance with supervision of residents ($N = 6$). One or two operators also mentioned assistance with meal preparation, activities and entertainment for residents, home repair, yard work, caring for hair and nails of residents, and direct health care. Staff were evidently providing a wide range of services, with few requiring high-level skills.

The duration of these staffing arrangements varied widely, from only a few months to those lasting five to ten years or more. Operators were asked to rate the helpfulness of staffers (as well as others providing support to them—see chap. 6) on a scale ranging from +3 ("the greatest possible help") to −3 ("makes more work for the operator"). Most of the staffers received strongly positive evaluations (+2 or +3), with only two of the fifty-six staff persons described as "making more work" for the operator.

Aside from the staff and the operator's kin who are living in the board-and-care households, there was often traffic through the home, including the operator's children, grandchildren, siblings, neighbors, and friends. Visitors also included the family and friends of the residents and various service providers. The homes were not closed environments and, as we will see (chaps. 5 and 6), often included both visitors and professionals coming in and excursions for the residents outside the home.

Privacy and Sharing of Space in the Home

Interviewers reported a wide array of physical configurations within the homes that were studied. One pivotal issue in how life flows through these homes is how (and by whom) the physical spaces are used. There are disagreements about the relative advantages of having more shared or more private space available in terms of privacy and interpersonal dynamics in the homes (Newman 1989). In both states, the operators were questioned about the degree to which physical space and amenities were shared by them, their families (if present in the household), and the residents of the home. Understanding how the operator, residents, and any coresiding kin of the operator collectively use space in the home illuminates the processes involved in providing care and the manner in which paying residents are or are not integrated into the social life of the home (see also chap. 6).

In terms of common space, residents and operators shared living space in the vast majority of homes in Baltimore (91.2 percent), with such joint use reported in three-quarters of homes operated by whites and all of the homes operated by African Americans. Separate living areas for residents were, however, significantly more likely to be found in homes with four or more residents (46.7 percent vs. 15.5 percent in smaller homes). This sharing of space enables joint activities and ongoing interactions among the residents as well as with the operators and their family members in the household. Separate spaces, while perhaps providing more quiet and privacy (Reschovsky and Ruchlin 1993), risk isolation of residents from the familial exchanges typical of those using joint living areas. The interviewer in one seven-resident home described having seen clients frequently walking through the living room, sitting on the porch, patio, or deck, and sitting in the dining room. Another operator talked a great deal about her coresiding granddaughter's involvement with the clients. This granddaughter woke up one confused client each morning and encouraged her to eat while at their common breakfast table. Such opportunities for interaction may not be suitable or preferable for all residents. Nor is such sharing always without problems. Another operator reported feeling very limited in her home by the presence of residents in the common living area. She could not watch television after 8:00 P.M., because to do so might disturb the clients when they retired to their rooms on the same floor. "I couldn't watch TV because they were all in bed, but I didn't want to go to bed myself."

Another indicator of the extent to which space is shared is the use of bathrooms. Most operators reported joint use of bathrooms by the residents, coresiding family members, and themselves, again with the pattern of common use more prevalent for African American operators (78.7 percent vs. 53.6 percent among white operators). It remains a possibility that there is greater sharing of physical space in the Baltimore homes operated by African Americans because of economic disadvantage, resulting in a smaller home with fewer bathrooms and less living space available to all. Examination of the Cleveland data, however, shows no difference by operator race in the numbers of bedrooms available for residents in their homes, arguing against this hypothesis.

The picture that emerges is one in which the residents are typically not segregated from the operator or the daily routine of the home in any meaningful way. They seem to be well integrated into the ebb and flow of everyday events. The outcomes of this common physical environment for collective activities and social relations in the homes are described in chapter 6.

There are other important indicators of the mutual use of the environment. Among Cleveland-area operators, 61.9 percent reported that residents of the home were allowed to use the kitchen. Questions of Baltimore operators further detailed this finding (see fig. 5). While most operators permit residents to have access to the refrigerator and/or food cupboards (peaking among homes with white operators and those charging higher fees), fewer operators permitted use of the stove (15.4 percent). This restriction may be related to realistic safety concerns about fires or burns, especially in homes containing one or more mentally ill or cognitively impaired individuals. Even "assisted living" facilities, which include access to the stove and refrigerators as part of their desired amenities, often

The Board-and-Care Environment □ 35

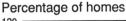

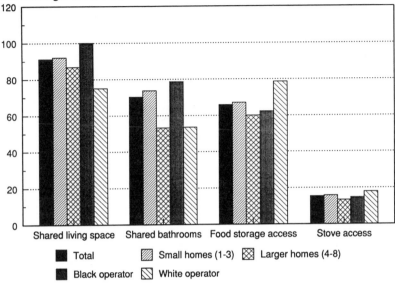

Fig. 5. Space and Access Issues in Baltimore Board-and-Care Homes

do not provide such access or actively forbid it (Kane, Wilson, and Clemmer 1993; Wilson 1993).

One operator reported locking the refrigerator at night, because, according to the interviewer, "she did not feel she could trust clients to stay out of the refrigerator, especially those who were on special diets." Similarly, another operator reported that mentally impaired clients wasted food by "taking bites out of it, squeezing eggs, and poking holes in things and then putting it back in the refrigerator." Another home operator with residents suffering from Alzheimer's disease and mental illness commented, "My kitchen is mine! I don't let anyone touch my pots and pans. I don't want them playing with food in my refrigerator. I don't know where their hands have been."

In both Cleveland and Baltimore, operators encouraged or allowed residents to bring their own belongings into the home when they arrived, rather than furnishing everything for the residents. Responses from residents of the homes in Cleveland showed that 87.2 percent had brought personal belongings to the home. Items brought most commonly included clothing, pictures, and small appliances (e.g., TV or radio). But a wide variety of other items, including furniture, hobby materials, and even small pets, were listed as having come with the residents to their new board-and-care environments. In many homes in the Baltimore area, the operators invited the interviewers to see the residents' rooms, proud of the physical environment they were able to offer to dependent adults in their care. In many instances, interviewers described how the rooms were personalized with photos and other mementoes, reducing the risk of an "institutional" feel in the board-and-care home. Another operator emphasized personalizing the space of clients. "I tell them if they got something that is theirs, then put it out so they can see it. This is their home—their room!"

Another noninstitutional aspect of the small board-and-care environment is the relatively high percentage of homes in Baltimore (64.8 percent) in which residents have single bedrooms. Reschovsky and Ruchlin (1993) used the percentage of single-occupancy bedrooms as an indicator of quality for the space and privacy dimension in their analysis of larger homes. Single bedrooms were more often reported by operators affiliated with Project HOME, since it was a program requirement, but the difference from nonparticipating homes was not statistically significant. The substantial percentage of single bedrooms reported here stands in contrast to research on larger homes, where double (or larger) rooms are the norm (Dittmar et al. 1983; Kane, Wilson, and Clemmer 1993; Mor, Sherwood, and Gutkin 1986). Although such configurations of single resident rooms are somewhat less common in the larger (four- to eight-resident) homes (46.7 percent), most residents in the Baltimore homes had their own bedrooms. This allowed a meaningful sense of privacy and some control over one's environment not typically found in larger, more institutional settings. One operator in Baltimore, whose house was described as clean, but with old and worn furnishings, told about Mr. T. and his room. She reported that Mr. T. collected everything and lined it up on his dresser. Although it was neat, according to the operator, it was all junk. Occasionally she tried to get into the room to clean it up, but he barred her from the room. According to the operator, he said, "This is my room. You can't come in here." Such situations clearly would not be tolerated in a more institutional setting. Even in board-and-care, this situation presents an ethical dilemma regarding the privacy of the resident versus the right to access by the home's operator. In many other settings, the residents' right to privacy would quickly give way to the organization's rules and its responsibility to protect them from anything that might harm them, resolving the dilemma in favor of the power of the institution. In board-and-care, however, the operator decides whether such situations are tolerable on a case-by-case basis.

There are, however, rules for the residents about access to particular spaces in many of the small board-and-care homes. Nearly half of Baltimore homes (47.8 percent) had some rules regarding room access, with the

existence of rules about evenly spread across homes of various sizes, operator race, and fee levels. Responses to questions asked of the operators
identified the rooms to which rules applied as mostly the operator's and
residents' bedrooms. Typically other persons (e.g., other residents or operator kin) were not allowed in these rooms without permission from their
occupants. Although reports from interviewers suggested that residents
could not lock the doors to their rooms for reasons of safety or regulations,
many operators (56 percent) reported that their residents had a lockable
storage area for personal belongings.

Our findings suggest that most small board-and-care homes demonstrate a physical environment that has been described as "familylike" or
"homelike" for residents (see also chap. 6) (Sherman and Newman 1988;
Eckert, Namazi, and Kahana 1987; Skruch 1993). While space and facilities
are regularly shared, there are usually some rules about privacy and access
to particular areas. This joint use of living space distinguishes the small
board-and-care homes we studied from the proposed standards for assisted living, where private living spaces with kitchenettes and lockable
doors have been proposed as the preferred options (Wilson 1993).

Control and Autonomy among Home Residents

One typical loss for individuals moving into an institutional setting, such
as a nursing home, is the autonomy to make decisions for themselves over
a variety of daily life issues. In nursing homes, for example, people are
awakened, fed, bathed, and given therapy on a tightly fixed schedule not
of their own choosing. They have little say in what they eat or with whom
they share space or activities (Diamond 1990). In contrast, resident choice,
independence, and mutual responsibility for the fulfillment of regular
tasks and activities (e.g., household work and rule setting) are key to the
emerging philosophy of assisted living (Mollica et al. 1992). Moon (1989)
and Newman (1989) both suggest that choice and flexibility for residents
are central to quality in board-and-care.

To assess the level of control in the lives of residents of small board-and-
care homes, two series of questions were included in the interviews with
operators in Cleveland, and related questions were asked in the fourth
interview of Baltimore operators. The results from the first set are summarized in figure 6. The responses detail an environment with more control
and autonomy for residents than is found in most formal organizations
providing care to dependent adults.

In the first series of questions operators were asked whether there were
"house rules" for residents concerning a variety of behaviors and activities

Percentage of homes

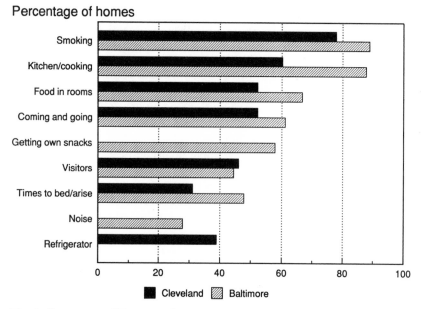

Fig. 6. Percentage of Homes with "House Rules" in Specific Areas

in the home. More home operators in Baltimore than in Cleveland reported rules in every category that matched between the two locations, but their relative rank was almost identical across both cities. Rules most commonly found in both studies pertained to smoking and to cooking food, again both activities that created potential fire risks when dealing with mentally and cognitively disabled residents. Operators had designated smoking areas or times, while some homes avoided the issue altogether by not accepting residents who smoked. One interviewer described a Baltimore operator who took great pride in her client's smoking area. "It was a small hall located off the main first floor hallway. It contained a chair, a small dresser, pictures, etc. Since she was told she had to have a designated smoking area, she did not want her client to feel isolated and made a very serious attempt to make the area one the client would enjoy."

Cooking food without supervision was often forbidden, and this prohibition was somewhat more common among African American operators in Baltimore. Having food in one's bedroom and "self service" of snacks also prompted rules in most Baltimore homes, with fewer restrictions on food in bedrooms in Cleveland homes. In Cleveland, African American operators were more likely to report rules regarding visiting hours (60 percent) and food in bedrooms (77.1 percent) than were white operators (39 percent and 40.3 percent, respectively) (see fig. 6). Lower-fee homes in that sample were also significantly more likely to have rules regarding food in bedrooms (63.6 percent vs. 39.6 percent in high-fee homes).

Interestingly, the "going to bed and getting-up times" item found fewer than half of Baltimore homes and only one-quarter of Cleveland homes reporting rules. But rules on this issue were significantly more common in larger Baltimore homes. While more of the homes had rules about coming and going, such rules were more common for African American operators. Fewer than half of homes had rules regarding visitors for the residents. On balance, the homes seem to be somewhat less rule-bound than many other long-term care facilities. This conclusion is further supported by data from Cleveland residents, where 93.1 percent of those surveyed responded negatively to a question asking them if there were rules in the home that they didn't like.

Many of the rules found in these homes are probably not unlike rules in families, where parents wish to know when a child is leaving the home and may restrict food in bedrooms. The small board-and-care homes appear to be less likely to have written rules than are most formal organizations, again acting more like families. Rules were typically unwritten, according to our interviewers. New residents would be informed of rules, with regular reinforcements for those with mental illness or cognitive limitations. Operators held the power of eviction for the most serious rule violators, where consistent behavior problems created danger or disruption to the operator or other residents (see also chap. 5). Less serious offenses could result in smaller sanctions (e.g., withholding dessert for a resident who refused to come out of her room to eat). Like families, then, rules were promulgated and enforced informally, with only extreme cases resulting in relocation of the troublesome resident.

The second area of questioning focused on aspects of home operation in which the residents might have some meaningful input to enhance their quality of life. Baltimore operators were asked whether "clients have any say in" a variety of decisions in the home. In Cleveland, a similar set of items was used, but operators were asked "Who usually makes the major decisions" in each of several designated areas. Findings are contrasted in table 1.

The great majority of Baltimore operators said that they took into account residents' preferences in the "kinds of food they eat." Resident input was also sought regarding the daily routine or schedule in the home and choices in coming and going from the home. In both of these latter areas, white operators were more likely to report giving their residents say in the decisions. Fewer homes allowed resident input in several other key areas, however. Residents were typically not consulted about whether another

Table 1

Resident Input into Decisions in Board-and-Care Homes

	Percentage of Homes in Which	
Issue	Operator Makes Major Decisions	Clients Have Input
Kinds of foods they eat	97.1	85.6
Setting meal times	93.5[a]	34.4
Changing bedrooms	88.2	32.2[b]
When someone must move out	84.6	39.1
Daily routine/schedule	NA	80.0[b]
Setting visiting hours	68.9[a]	54.4
Coming and going	39.6	77.8[b]

Note: Data in column 1 are from Cleveland ($N = 136$), data in column 2 are from Baltimore ($N = 90$).
[a]Difference by size is statistically significant ($p < .05$).
[b]Difference by race is statistically significant ($p < .05$.)

resident must move out, meal times, or changing of bedrooms by residents. In most homes, these were decisions that operators retained, in consultation with the resident involved, his or her kin, and appropriate social service providers. These gatekeeping functions (Bernstein 1982) were primarily the responsibility of operators in these homes, as they are for the administrators in larger facilities.

Examining the responses from Cleveland, however, points up a different dimension of these decision-making processes (see table 1). While the responses from Baltimore operators emphasized that residents do have input, the Cleveland operators reinforced the notion that final decision making typically rests with them. With one exception (coming and going from the home), operators defined themselves as the major decision makers in most areas, a definition consistent with their responsibility for care of others in the home. This was especially the case in larger homes for rules about setting meal times (100 percent said operators were decision makers, compared with 89.9 percent in smaller homes) and visiting hours (81.6 percent of operators defined themselves as the decision maker, compared with 61.6 percent in smaller homes), where operators from larger homes were significantly more likely to make these decisions.

While these homes clearly did not provide residents with the same level of autonomy and control that would be found in their own homes and apartments, operators made efforts to solicit input in several key areas and seemed to limit rule making to issues having to do with the safety and comfort of multiple unrelated adults sharing a living environment. The rules seemed less restrictive than those typical of nursing homes, and clients, by virtue of participation in decisions that shaped their day-to-day lives, had levels of autonomy more akin to those in current assisted-living settings (Kane, Wilson, and Clemmer 1993). Operators probably could not manage their homes if they had a policy of total autonomy, especially given the mental illnesses and cognitive impairments that often prompt placement in such a home in the first place (see chap. 6).

Services and Equipment Available in Homes

The Service Package

Although there are a number of ways in which these homes resemble families, they are, nevertheless, intended to provide some level of service to physically and mentally impaired adults. Prior research (Dittmar et al. 1983; Mor, Sherwood, and Gutkin 1986) and recommendations by experts (Scanlon and Feder 1983) argue that residential care facilities, including board-and-care homes, should offer a wide range of services to their clients. There is some debate regarding the level of services in contemporary board-and-care homes, with some authors (Kane, Wilson, and Clemmer 1993) suggesting that these homes are restricted to the provision of housing, meals, and protective oversight. They maintain that assisted living, in contrast to board-and-care, provides a wider range of services, including assistance in the performance of activities of daily living, coupled with the capacity to meet needs for "unscheduled assistance." This service provision criterion is the crux of Kane and associates' definitional distinction between board-and-care and assisted living (1993, 1). According to Kane and associates (1993, 2) "these [board-and-care] homes do not offer a comprehensive range of services or claim an ability to meet unscheduled needs." In contrast with this view, however, the services we expected to find in the small homes are those often described in conjunction with assisted living, including personal care, assistance with medications, housekeeping, shopping, meals, laundry, transportation, and so-cial/recreational services (Mollica et al. 1992).

In both Cleveland and Baltimore, responding operators were asked whether they provided a range of services (or arranged to have others provide them, in Baltimore) for residents in their homes on a regular basis. The results for Baltimore are profiled in figure 7.

Eleven of the sixteen services we listed were provided in at least 90 percent of Baltimore-area board-and-care homes. Most common were assistance with medications, three meals per day and snacks, laundry, trans-

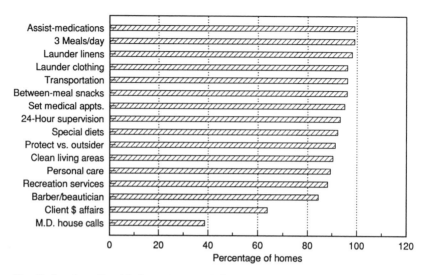

Fig. 7. Services Provided or Arranged for Residents by Home Operators in Baltimore

portation, twenty-four-hour supervision, and cleaning. Only one of the services, arranging visits by the doctor to the board-and-care home, was provided by fewer than half of operators. But even this service was available in nearly two-thirds of the larger (four to eight resident) homes in the Baltimore sample (see fig. 7). Nine of these items were mirrored in the Cleveland study, with strikingly similar percentages of operators responding positively for most. In only two cases, providing transportation (76.3 percent) and arranging medical appointments (71.9 percent), were Cleveland operators substantially *less* likely to provide the comparable services than were their Baltimore counterparts.

Comparisons across differing home and operator characteristics revealed a relatively high level of consistency. White operators were somewhat less likely to provide laundry services, higher-fee homes more often provided barber and beautician services, and more higher-fee homes claimed that they acted to protect their residents from outsiders who might bother or take advantage of them. For the remaining services, the differences between groups were not significant, and often the differences were very small indeed. The levels of services offered in these homes, at least in terms of the questions we asked, were high and surprisingly consistent.

When we asked Baltimore operators what other services they provided, answers included such options as shopping for the clients, acting as a liaison with the resident's family, and organizing or arranging religious services. Operators appeared to view the service package in their homes as rather flexible and adaptable to the needs of those they housed. Some operators simply informed us that what their work involved was "whatever the clients need." If this criterion was actually in force in many small homes, their service provision met or exceeded that described for assisted living settings by Kane and associates (1993). This also raises the troubling issue of whether operators, by being willing to do whatever was needed, are able to recognize appropriate limits on their ability to provide care. The issue of whether operators become overloaded by demands for care by multiply disabled persons aging in place is discussed further in chapter 4.

Specialized Equipment

Another way to evaluate the services available to the residents of small board-and-care homes is to examine the types of specialized equipment and safety features intended to assist physically impaired residents with their everyday routines. An inventory of possible equipment was presented to the Baltimore operators to determine how many homes were equipped with each item. Some of these items designed to enhance safety, such as handrails on all staircases, were to be found in almost all (88.9 percent) of the homes. Most homes also had grab-bars (72.2 percent) and antiskid runners (90.0 percent) in their bathtubs to assist residents, with grab-bars more prevalent in higher-fee homes (84.1 percent).

Certain pieces of equipment were found more frequently in larger (four- to eight-resident) homes. For example, both wheelchair-accessible toilets (71.4 percent compared with 42.1 percent; 46.7 percent overall in the sample) and specialized toilet chairs or seats (71.4 percent compared with 38.2 percent; 43.3 percent overall in the sample) were more common in homes with four or more residents. Hospital-type adjustable beds were found more often (39.3 percent) in homes operated by whites than in those with African American operators (16.7 percent; 23.9 percent overall in the sample). Other devices, such as elevators or chair lifts on stairs (4.4 percent) or wheelchair lifts (1.1 percent) were found infrequently in the small board-and-care homes studied.

It is perhaps surprising that there were not larger differences in equipment by the average level of fees paid by the residents, since higher income should have enabled operators to purchase more specialized equipment. In addition, prior research (Sherwood, Mor, and Gutkin 1981) had suggested that homes charging higher rates tended to accept more physically impaired residents. However, both of those results ignored the issue of *need* and the higher reimbursement rate for mentally ill individuals housed in the Baltimore-area board-and-care homes under Project HOME. While all of the homes studied in Baltimore had at least one older adult receiving care, many of the other residents were dependent because they were mentally ill or cognitively impaired (see chap. 5). For those individuals, the physical appliances and equipment in our questions were generally unnecessary. It is therefore difficult to fault operators who lacked equipment, since in many cases this absence did not reflect unmet needs, but instead, a lack of need for such supports.

Quality of the Physical Environment

Since much of the literature and public knowledge about board-and-care homes is negative, we decided to evaluate the quality of the homes and the care given in them in several ways. The first way was to examine the quality of the physical environment. Given the reports of poor environmental quality in board-and-care homes (as described in chap. 1), evaluation of the physical environment in such small homes is important for the development of appropriate public policy in this area. Reschovsky and Ruchlin (1993) evaluated the facility environment in board-and-care homes in terms of noise, odor, illumination, clutter, wall cleanliness, the condition of furniture, and the presence of windows. Overall, they found that these environmental indicators were better in nonprofit homes. Little additional *systematic* evaluation has been made of the physical environment of board-and-care homes.

In the Cleveland study, interviewers were asked to rate a set of environmental traits at the conclusion of the resident interviews. Results showed that in a strong majority of homes, interviewers rated the condition of the walls/flooring and the furniture as good or excellent (81.7 percent for each). Most (83.0 percent) reported the staff to be "nearly constantly available" to residents. In several questions on the neatness, lighting, odors, and noise, most homes were placed in the highest category (85.8 percent neat, 60.6 percent ample lighting, 96.3 percent having no odors, and 70.2 percent quiet).

As part of the fourth and final interviews with Baltimore operators, we asked the interviewers to rate the quality of ten aspects of the physical environment of the home on a four-point rating scale (4 = excellent).

Figure 8 summarizes these ratings, comparing homes by race of the operator; some significant differences emerged. We were surprised to see that so few of these homes were rated by the interviewers (all mature, middle-class women) as "poor" or even "fair." These two categories combined never exceeded one home in six on any of the ten aspects of the physical environment evaluated, and on some (e.g., operator availability to residents, excess noise) none of the homes were rated as "poor." Be-

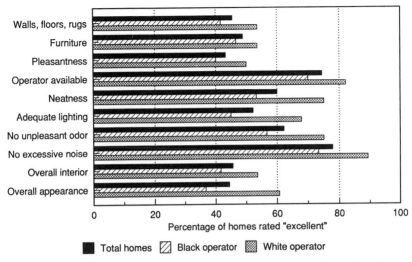

Fig. 8. Interviewer Ratings of Home Quality in Baltimore Board-and-Care Homes

cause of the skewed distributions of responses, the "excellent" category was compared with the other three and is reported in the figure. Excellent ratings were common; between 43 percent and 77 percent of homes rated as "excellent" on each of the ten interviewer ratings items used. There were some differences by home size (data not shown), but none of the differences were statistically significant, and the direction varied. More of the smaller homes, for example, had excellent ratings for pleasantness and furnishings, among other aspects, but "larger" (four- to eight-resident) homes received more "excellent" rankings on the availability of the home's operator to the clients and absence of noise (see fig. 8).

Homes operated by whites generally ranked somewhat higher than those of African Americans on most of these items, although for only two items (adequacy of lighting and overall appearance) did the difference reach statistical significance. Once again, differences may have more to do with economic factors, with African American operators operating lower-cost homes (see chap. 3). Higher fees should enable operators to provide a higher quality physical environment. As expected, homes charging higher fees to their residents (data not shown) did score more excellent rankings from interviewers on the ten aspects of the physical environment rated. Although none of the differences were statistically significant, they are all in the expected direction, with higher-fee homes more often scored as excellent than lower-fee homes. Our findings support contentions (Lyon 1993; Newman 1989) that some aspects of quality are linked to higher fees.

Interviewer comments included descriptions of some homes as "immaculate," or "well-kept." Not unusual was a description of a well-run home in which "all rooms are kept clean daily, are comfortably furnished, bright, and include radios, TV sets, and wall-to-wall carpet. Bathrooms are on the same level, and an enclosed sun porch has been added for clients' comfort." Another operator had renovated an old row house in one of the highest crime areas of the city, which our interviewer described as "lovely . . . you can't believe your eyes." One operator, describing her philosophy to the interviewer, said, "One person can't move the world, but that person can make a difference. Around here, I keep my sidewalk clean and my place looking good. The kids ring my doorbell to give me pieces of paper, because they know I keep my place clean."

Interviewer descriptions such as the following were common. "The home is a townhouse located in (neighborhood). The home is well-kept. The yard and porch are filled with flowers. The downstairs furnishings are old and worn, but the home is neat and clean. Probably due to the dark furnishings and the paneled walls, the rooms downstairs are not well lit. The three bedrooms upstairs each contain a set of twin beds and two dressers. The rooms are brighter here, and this is where the clients sleep. Personal things of the clients were noted all about the room (posters, pictures, stuffed animals, etc.)."

High general ratings should not disguise the fact that some homes in our samples had questionable physical environments that would probably cause negative reactions from regulators. One home, for example, was described by the interviewer as "not particularly clean, and roaches were present on the first two visits." Another home was described as "clean—but cluttered—just filled with memorabilia." Others found "a slight urine odor" and rooms that seemed "lived in." In another case, a home run by a man was "comfortably furnished but cluttered. Dust was noted on the furniture and dishes were on the counter and in the sink. However, there was no indication that what was noted in the home was other than what would be found in another family home." In another case a description said, "The home is in disrepair on a small, quiet street. Furniture was worn, the walls were grayish white from dirt and grime, and the rooms within my eyesight were small." While these descriptions are undesirable, they are far from the worst-case conditions described in some other reports. It remains a possibility, however, that operators with homes in more questionable physical shape simply refused our interviews for fear of negative consequences. In sum, the conditions we found were not unlike housing conditions typical of their neighborhoods and socioeconomic peers, ranging from immaculate to poorly managed, much as would be the case for family households.

Community Acceptance

A major concern of many facilities caring for dependent adults is the so-called NIMBY syndrome (not in my backyard). This syndrome involves community resistance to the care of specialized populations in their neighborhoods, often based on fears of unusual behaviors or diminished property values (Sherman and Newman 1988). This syndrome is most likely to appear in resistance to the opening or development of new facilities to care for specialized populations (e.g., deinstitutionalized mentally ill, physically or developmentally disabled) in a residential neighborhood. According to research (Mangum 1985), these fears are greater with young, mentally disabled or ill persons than they are with the elderly. The social marginality of residents may be responsible for some of the discomfort and lack of community acceptance associated with this syndrome. The negative community reaction may be lessened, however, when homes are small and unobtrusive (Sherman and Newman 1988).

Since the small homes we studied often shelter both mentally ill and elderly individuals, the NIMBY syndrome is a risk they may face. With only limited information regarding the community acceptance of small homes from Sherman and Newman (1988), Baltimore operators were asked a series of questions on community acceptance in the fourth interview. The results were somewhat surprising.

Three-quarters of the operators reported that "most" of their neighbors were aware that they were providing board-and-care services in their homes, a result that was consistent across all groups of operators. Very few (4.5 percent) admitted having avoided informing those in their communities about the work they were doing. One operator expressed concern, stating that she didn't "advertise" what she does. According to her account, she kept clients from sitting where neighbors could see what they were doing. "Sometimes they talk to themselves or do strange things. I don't let them talk to the neighbors other than to say hello. . . . I lost my last home because the landlord didn't want any 'nuts' living in his house." Overall, few of the operators appeared to be concerned about the potential for negative reactions of those living around them. Slightly over half (53.4 percent) had received some sort of reaction from neighbors to their caregiving work, especially white operators. These reactions were, however, predominantly positive (87.2 percent), with almost all African American operators (96.3 percent) reporting that any reactions they received were "mostly good."

In addition, most could identify no memorable event, either positive or negative, involving neighbors or groups in their communities. Although we expected that Project HOME residences would be more publicly known, there were no differences from nonaffiliated homes on any of these community reaction variables.

Specific examples of reactions from the community focused mostly on negative events. One home operator reported to the interviewer that over the years, from time to time, she had had slight difficulty with neighbors who are not quite comfortable with having her operate a board-and-care home. A male operator in Baltimore, who admittedly "kept a low profile" about his home, was surprised to receive positive comments about one of his clients being a "sweet man" who spent time with neighborhood children, pushing them on the swings. Yet when another of his neighbors discovered his board-and-care home, she organized a meeting of the civic association, where that same operator was asked rudely whether his residents would defecate on the lawn or undress outside. At that meeting, he agreed to house only women, because of concern about potential child molestation expressed by those present at the meeting. Such discomfort from neighbors, however, appeared to trouble the minority of operators. Although some of the homes were undoubtedly operating without the knowledge of some in their immediate surroundings (i.e., neighbors, community associations), it was clear from these responses that most operators have not suffered significant negative reactions.

There are several potential explanations for these findings and differences. First, small homes such as those we studied may not trigger the same level of community reaction as a larger, more institutional setting might. Second, the fact that many of the operators had been members of these communities for years prior to starting to provide care to dependent adults may act to minimize neighbors' fears of the unknown associated with a newly established facility. In addition, many of the homes were located in poorer neighborhoods that may be less capable of organizing effective resistance or may simply be more permissive. Such areas are justifiably more concerned with the pressing urban issues of crime, poverty, and drug abuse than they are with the presence of small board-and-care homes in their midst.

□ SMALL BOARD-AND-CARE HOMES reflect social marginality in their environments in a variety of ways. They walk a fine line between family and business, primary and formal groups, public and private organizations. In many ways, the evolution of board-and-care homes as a grass-roots approach to dealing with displaced and dependent adults has meant that operators of homes could largely define the parameters and the context for interaction in ways that suited their situations, the needs of their families, the needs of other clients, and the physical constraints imposed by the structure of the home.

Homes we studied typically involved public living spaces shared by operators (and their families) and residents, with rules over use of space that are unwritten and akin to those that would be imposed by families with small children who might get into trouble with fire or access to the food supplies. Since many of the homes are typical family homes, with limited modifications, sharing of space and facilities is natural. While some operators did separate their living space from that of their residents (e.g., bedrooms and a sitting room on a separate floor), such arrangements were not the norm. Descriptions of comings and goings by residents and their kin, pets, children, and extended kin of the operator were common in our interviewers' observations in these homes.

A certain amount of privacy and control is available to residents in the homes. Although the operator still held a position of power relative to the residents in many ways, most residents had private rooms, which they were usually encouraged to decorate and furnish with their own belongings. Most had a lockable storage space for personal items, even though doors to rooms were not lockable for safety reasons. Rules for behavior were not seen as onerous, and residents were even given some say in decisions regarding their day-to-day lives. This stands in sharp contrast to the situation of older adults in nursing homes, where meal times are regimented and decisions are often driven by staffing and medical requirements, rather than preferences of the residents (Diamond 1990).

Services also reflected those that would typically occur within the family context, ranging from personal care to transportation and recreation. The statements of many operators that they did "whatever the clients need" reflect a global and individualistic approach to care, contrasted to the constrained and medical nature of care provided in most formal organizations providing long-term health care. Operators did not place limits around the tasks they might perform, although there were often legal limits (e.g., administering medications) to which they must be sensitive (Kane, Wilson, and Clemmer 1993; Moon 1989). Nurse aides or home health aides, by contrast, have specific services they are permitted to provide to their clients or patients, dictated by rules of the organizations that employ them.

We were surprised to learn that few Baltimore operators had experienced negative reactions from neighbors regarding the care provided to dependent, often cognitively or mentally impaired, residents. While some noted taking care to avoid difficulties, as had the adult foster care providers studied by Sherman and Newman (1988), others suggested support for their efforts among neighbors in their communities. Whether the nature of the neighborhoods themselves (or absence of a "neighborhood" in the case of some rural homes) or the operator's prior tenure in the community muted the resistance often seen to the placement of new care facilities is a remaining empirical question.

Overall, the quality of the physical environment in the homes we studied in both locations was good, suggesting that the negative discussions of board-and-care homes are overblown or selective in their views. Like prior research (Dittmar 1989, 3), our research did not find "board and care homes to be abusive or life threatening." Although there may have been bad homes that refused our interviews, as other researchers have noted (Dittmar 1989), it must be emphasized that there are also high-quality homes available. The physical environments were rated by our interviewers as good to excellent on most key dimensions of quality (Newman 1989).

Small board-and-care homes, then, provide a unique setting for caring for adults with moderate levels of dependency who do not require medical care. The physical environment reflects many of the quasi-familial aspects that have been noted as desirable for individuals requiring custodial care (Kane, Wilson, and Clemmer 1993). As we shall see in coming chapters, this setting provides a context for social interaction that is quite distinct from the formal institutional settings in which medical care is provided.

3 □ The Economics of Small Board-and-Care Homes

□ ISSUES AND concerns related to economics have been at the forefront of debates regarding board-and-care services. On the institutional level, debates over mechanisms for providing reimbursement for custodial care of dependent adult populations (i.e., care beyond the medical model services that are now publicly financed) remain unresolved. Ensuring a continuing supply of care providers through adequate financing is critical to maintaining an adequate number of board-and-care facilities nationally (Conley 1989; Dittmar 1989; Harmon 1982). Some authors (Mor, Sherwood, and Gutkin 1986; Stone and Newcomer 1986) point out that fees and the underlying reimbursement systems largely responsible for them are currently set too low to encourage new operators to enter the field or to permit upgrading the existing stock of homes. Thus, both the survival and the quality of board-and-care services turn on economic issues.

On the operators' level, concerns about the adequacy of income from fees, the coverage for additional expenses associated with providing services, and the financial ability to continue operating a board-and-care home all are central issues. Residents (or potential residents) face uncertainty as to whether their resources will be sufficient to purchase board-and-care services of good quality (Ehrlich 1986). Indeed, board-and-care homes have been referred to as "life care communities for the poor," given the disadvantaged financial status of the bulk of their clientele (Moon 1989, viii). Other authors and researchers (Ehrlich 1986; Eckert, Namazi, and Kahana 1987; Dobkin 1989; Moon 1989) have described the relatively low reimbursement rates and the fact that the clientele of board-and-care homes has largely constituted an underclass of the dependent adult/elderly population. Although, for the most part, public funds do not pay directly for board and care services, the federal Supplemental Security Income (SSI) program, supplemented by many states, effectively pays for these services for most low-income residents. Public and media concerns focus on whether public funds are, in fact, being well-spent on safe, quality environments and whether cost savings could be attained through changes in the programs housing dependent populations.

The research on economic issues related to board-and-care has, to date, primarily focused on the organizational-level debate, describing the federal funding mechanisms and the state-level subsidies offered in many locations (CSSP 1988). The heavy reliance on SSI and Social Security retirement or disability benefits as mechanisms of funding (via the individual recipient) are well known (Capitman 1989; Ehrlich 1986). According to a recent report (Hawes et al. 1993), forty states and the District of Columbia provide state supplementation to SSI for *some* recipients in board-and-care homes or similar settings. Such supplements enable individuals who do not qualify for nursing homes and need no medical services to meet their dependency needs related to activities of daily living by purchasing services, often in a residential setting such as a board-and-care home (Capitman 1989; CSSP 1988).

Although there has been some mixed success in redirecting funds designated for medical care to board-and-care homes, often under the rubric of Medicaid 2176 waivers (see Capitman 1989; Feder et al. 1989), finding additional sources of financing for this dependent population to purchase the care they require has not been systematically addressed in public policy (Capitman 1989). The fact that the populations housed in small board-and-care homes relate to a variety of agencies and reimbursement systems (those pertaining to aging, health, physical disabilities, developmental disabilities, and mental illness, among others) on state and federal levels means that financing these homes is everyone's problem and no one's responsibility (Baggett 1989).

One commonly voiced concern is that the quality of care is linked to the amount of money paid for that care (CSSP 1988; Newman 1989; Reschovsky and Ruchlin 1993). Thus, when reports of poor care are heard, it is often assumed that adequate financing will resolve all of the problems. Indeed, some research has positively linked aspects of care quality to the fees being paid (Lyon 1993), but the difficulty with evaluating quality of care has limited research in this area (Reschovsky and Ruchlin 1993).

Ironically, those state subsidies that have their levels of reimbursement differentiated according to the amount of care required by the residents create some interesting dilemmas (Feder et al. 1989). Operators of board-and-care homes may try to hold vacant beds open for residents with the highest reimbursement rates (Dittmar 1989). Varying fees may actually create a financial disincentive to operators to do their best, since fees decline if the condition of residents in their care improves. It is, therefore, important to examine the small board-and-care homes that operate largely outside of the major reimbursement systems for medical care, to determine their financial health and stability as caregiving institutions. Ultimately, their fiscal condition frames the capacity of the operator to continue running the home, so that small board-and-care homes running at a deficit should be a cause for concern (Chen 1989).

In addition to this policy-level debate, relatively little attention has been given to the microeconomics of board-and-care homes. Chen (1989) reported that many of the homes he studied were just breaking even every month. Given the scanty information, many questions remain unanswered. How much do operators receive for the care they provide in these smaller homes? What are the sources of funding for resident fees? Are operators able to make ends meet on the funds they are receiving? How do operators view and manage the financial side of operating their homes?

The role of money and in fact the amounts received have been little understood in this environment. This chapter outlines in some detail the financial operation of the homes we studied in Baltimore, including fees from residents and their sources, the costs of home operation, the financial management by residents and operators, and the operators' views of the relative importance of money to their work. The complexity of these issues for the small homes will become apparent as the data are presented, as will the issues of economic marginality that place their continued operation at risk.

Since so little is known about the details of financial operations in these homes, this served as a central focus in our second interview with operators in Baltimore. These Baltimore data are supplemented by and compared with more limited data on this topic gathered several years earlier in the Cleveland area. Homes in both cities demonstrate diversity in their financial well-being and in how operators approach and manage the income and expenses of providing board-and-care services.

The Project HOME program, operating in Maryland, includes SSI supplementation at rates among the highest in the country at the time of our study in Maryland (see chap. 1; CSSP 1988; Dobkin 1989). As the following analyses show, supplements make some important differences in outcomes for residents, operators, and homes.

The economics of home operation demonstrate the same marginality that appears in other aspects of these small homes. The operators did not always distinguish funds for home operation from other funds coming into the household, nor did they expend them in ways to distinguish them from personal and family resources. The lines between board-and-care as "business" and as "family" appeared to be quite permeable in the areas of money and its management.

Income from Board-and-Care: Amounts and Sources

Prior research on board-and-care homes, emphasizing the larger facilities, has stressed the modest amounts that most residents pay for shelter and services (Mor, Gutkin, and Sherwood 1985). In our studies, the income from resident fees was one of the simplest items to document, because the operators appeared to be fairly certain about how much each resident was paying per month for housing, meals, and all of the other services provided. Few operators (four in the first interview in Baltimore) refused to report these figures, so the data are fairly complete. As the distributions in figure 9 demonstrate, the dollar figures that individual residents paid for their housing and care each month varied substantially. The operators in the Baltimore sample, reporting individually for each current client, said that about one in five was paying less than $400 monthly ($4800 annually) for housing, meals, and care. In fact, one individual was reported as paying nothing at the time of the first Baltimore interview. Over one-quarter of Cleveland operators (28.8 percent) reported *average* monthly fees in their homes to be in the same low range (i.e., less than $400 per month). These modest figures mirror those reported in a prior study by Mor and his associates (1985).

Although the distribution of operator-reported monthly fees is larger in Baltimore than in Cleveland (perhaps in part because in Baltimore we inquired about *individual* residents, rather than *averages* for all clients housed), 63.2 percent of the fees paid by residents in Baltimore and 82.7 percent of the reported averages for fees in Cleveland homes were under $1,000 per month. Obviously, this compares quite favorably with the fees

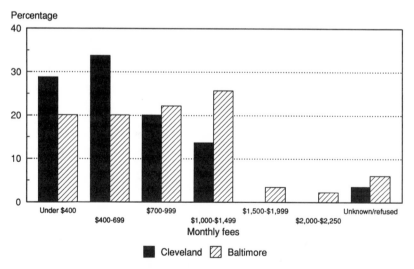

Fig. 9. Distribution of Resident Monthly Fees in Baltimore and Cleveland
Note: Fee values corrected to 1990 dollars using the Consumer Price Index.

being paid for higher-skilled nursing home care and equally skilled assisted living settings, signaling a potentially substantial cost saving for placing appropriate individuals in this lower-cost alternative (see also Feder et al. 1989; Kane, Wilson, and Clemmer 1993; Sherwood and Morris 1983; Sherwood, Morris, and Sherwood 1986). While a few Baltimore operators reported fees above $2,000 per month for their residents, overall, small board-and-care homes focus on the low-cost provision of services.

Sources of Variation in Fees

Fees vary both within and between homes. Both the characteristics of the residents and those of the home and its operator seem to influence the amount being charged for board-and-care services in particular situations.

There is often substantial variation *within* the homes in what particular resident/clients pay for services. Only 14.8 percent of the homes in Baltimore with two or more residents ($N = 81$) reported charging the same fees for all of the residents about whom data were collected. In general, these single-fee homes were smaller (two or three residents), since larger numbers of residents increased the likelihood that monthly fees would vary.

In several instances, each resident of the home paid a slightly different fee. One home, for example, reported four different fees for each of four residents, ranging from $352 to $567 per month. In many of these cases, however, the differences among the residents' fees within the homes were quite small (under $20). Other homes showed more extreme variation in what residents paid. For example, in one home one resident reportedly paid nothing, while two others paid $821 per month; in a second example, one resident paid $250, while the remaining three residents each paid $1,026.

Fees also vary in many of the homes participating in Project HOME, since the program subsidizes individual residents, rather than reimbursing homes across the board for all of their clients. In some homes, in which all residents were program participants, there was homogeneity in fees. Examples of the other extreme are two homes of three residents each: one in which two residents paid fees of $1,011, while a third paid $495, and a second in which one resident paid $979, while two others paid much lower fees ($472 and $475). This leaves open the possibility that Project HOME funds (and those of similar resident-based subsidies) may actually benefit other residents in homes participating in the program, a consequence not intended by the policymakers who established them.

Apparently, in these smaller homes, operators set fees somewhat flexibly, on a case-by-case basis. Sometimes attachment to a client prompts an operator to keep them for less than the "going rate." One Baltimore operator recounted keeping a man with limited financial resources for $400 per month, less than her usual rate. "The money doesn't matter. He is happy here and he's no trouble. He really isn't nursing home material yet." Given the diversity in fees within homes, the next logical question to ask is what factors or techniques determine the fees charged by the board-and-care home operators? How do operators set their fees?

There are a variety of possible ways in which operators may establish fees for their homes or for particular residents within them. Baltimore operators were asked, in an open-ended format, how they decided how much they got for each individual client each month. Many of the operators responded that their fees were set by programs to which they were affiliated, as has been the case in other research (Dittmar et al. 1983). Among operators in Baltimore, where a major state subsidy program (Project HOME) supports some elderly and dependent adults in board-and-care homes, 56.3 percent of operators said that their fees were set by what the program was willing to pay. But a variety of other factors also shape the amounts that are charged to residents, since not all homes participate in that program (or not all residents in a given home are subsidized by the program). For example, 11.7 percent of Baltimore operators set fees on the basis of the incomes or assets of their clients, 15.5 percent took the level of health problems (and consequent amount of work for themselves) into consideration, only 3.9 percent considered what other homes charged, 6.8 percent negotiated with the family or others regarding an appropriate fee, 6.8 percent had set fees that were adjusted for resident income, 2.9 percent reported that they knew from experience what to charge for a particular client, 2.9 percent based fees on costs for food, and 1.9 percent reported that they used some other means to establish appropriate costs. According to the operator of one Baltimore home, her rates were set by finding out what others charged, cutting those fees in half, and then making adjustments for what the resident's family could afford. In many cases ($N = 22$), operators reported more than one means of determining fees. This flexibility in setting fees, including consideration of ability to pay, has also been noted in prior studies of larger board-and-care homes (Dittmar et al. 1983).

Some systematic variations in fee levels were supported by the operator reports. Residents living in homes affiliated with the Project HOME program paid similar fees regardless of race (median: $964 for whites, $962 for African Americans). In nonparticipating homes, however, white residents paid significantly higher monthly fees (median, $923) than did their African American counterparts (median, $423). Females ($923) paid more than males ($702, not statistically significant); those under age forty-five paid significantly more ($727) than those between forty-five and sixty-four ($616), but less than residents over age sixty-five ($945). Residents who reported having some family members available to them also paid significantly higher fees, on average, than those without kin ($923 vs. $518).

There were also differences by traits of the home or operator. White operators charged significantly higher fees (median, $1,011) than did their African American counterparts (median, $616). Small homes of three or fewer residents charged only slightly less than larger ones, but the difference achieved statistical significance (median: $900, compared with $974). Again, this may be influenced by the size limitation on Project HOME facilities, pairing high subsidies with a limited number of residents permitted in each home.

Sources of Income to Residents

As has been shown in other studies (Capitman 1989; CSSP 1988; Dittmar et al. 1983), residents of board-and-care homes are typically receiving income from one or more public or programmatic sources. Among Baltimore home residents (according to operator reports), 32 percent received Social Security benefits, 12 percent received disability income, 43.7 percent received SSI, only 7.9 percent got a pension, 5.9 percent received Veteran's Administration benefits, 5.9 percent received income from savings or investments, 5 percent got income from their families, and 1.2 percent earned wages.

Data from Cleveland suggest a somewhat different profile, with 11.9 percent of residents reporting that they received SSI benefits and 34.4 percent reporting income from either Social Security retirement or disability programs. These differences may, in part, be due to different client characteristics in the two locations (partially related to the presence of the Project HOME program in Maryland), differences in the formats of the income questions, or the fact that operators reported in Baltimore, while only "able" residents were asked about income sources in Cleveland (see chap. 6). Significant reliance on SSI is not surprising, given other research emphasizing the importance of this income source in the board-and-care population (CSSP 1988; Capitman 1989).

Many residents received income from multiple sources. In Baltimore, for example, operators reported that 28.6 percent of residents were receiving income from two or more of the six specific sources of income about which we inquired (Social Security, SSI, disability of any type, savings or investments, wages, or their families). Not surprisingly, operators in Baltimore reported that two-thirds of those receiving SSI were receiving no other source of income. Operators also reported that one-fifth of residents either received income from none of the sources on our list or the sources of income to specific residents were unknown. This lack of knowledge is reinforced by data regarding residents' money management (discussed later in this chapter).

Given the types of sources under consideration, however, it is clear that most residents are poor or near-poor persons. Specifically, the largest source of income to the residents of small board-and-care home in Baltimore, as in some other studies, was SSI, the federal program mandated to support those elderly in the most vulnerable economic positions. Moreover, the fees paid to the operators and the homes' overall economic viability are shaped by the limited resources available to many of their current and potential clients.

Overall Income to the Home

How much did the homes collect per month from their residents, assuming that all anticipated fees were paid? Estimates of total income in Baltimore were based on data collected on a maximum of four residents for each home. In homes with five or more residents, each additional person was assumed to be paying the average fee for the first four residents, about whom data were collected. Figure 10 outlines monthly incomes to the homes from board-and-care services.

Home income from provision of board-and-care services ranged from $205 per month to $16,000 per month, with the median amount for all homes in Baltimore at $1,683 per month. Only four homes reported incomes totaling over $5,000 per month, with 83.7 percent reporting less than $3,000 per month in income from fees. As expected, homes with fewer than three residents had lower incomes from board-and-care services than did their larger counterparts. Whites reported larger incomes from operation of their homes than did African Americans, but the differences were not large and, in part, mirrored the variation in the number of residents being housed. The income stream from providing board-and-care services was higher to the homes affiliated with Project HOME (using the median dollar values). These average incomes from those participating and those not participating are more similar, however, than might have been expected. This may be because Project HOME, while providing a substantial financial subsidy, also limits the number of residents being cared for. Thus, even with higher per-resident fees for providing service, the income to the participating home is still fairly modest on average.

The fact that this difference is reversed when the mean is used as the measure of central tendency (i.e., higher *mean* income to nonparticipants in Project HOME) suggests that a few very high income homes that were not involved in the Project HOME program are pulling up the mean. These

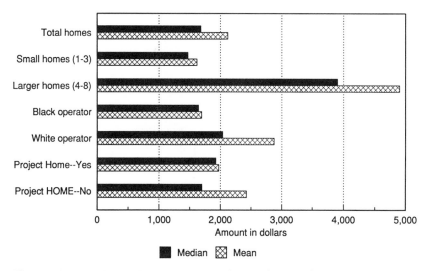

Fig. 10. Average Home Income per Month in Baltimore from Board-and-Care Services

Note: Fee data were collected on up to four residents in the first Baltimore interview. For larger homes, fees for additional residents were assumed to be the mean of the first four.

homes were part of a small group ($N = 4$ of Baltimore homes, whose median monthly fee to residents was $1500 or more, which might be called *financially elite*. These elite homes were private-pay with higher fee levels. Given their distinctiveness from the great majority of homes under examination, they are described separately, as a subset of the high-fee homes, in a later section of this chapter.

Overall, the operators of small board-and-care homes were not receiving large sums of money per month for the housing and care they provide. Small size and low per-resident fees did not add up to a substantial flow of income for most of the homes. The next issue to evaluate, then, is the expenses involved with operation of a home on a routine basis. To determine whether and when these homes are "profitable," it is necessary to compare the costs of providing the services to the income available to pay for these services.

Expenses: Expected and Unexpected

Chen (1989) suggests that expenses can be divided into start-up costs and operating expenses. As we have already seen (chap. 2), relatively few of the operators in the small homes we studied acquired properties to offer services. While many of them had made modifications, the median cost of such modifications was modest ($2,000). These start-up costs were undoubtedly minimized for our sample by the absence of regulations relating to structural features of the homes (e.g., corridor width requirements, chair lift to second floor), which could otherwise be quite costly to the operators in larger or licensed board-and-care homes (Chen 1989). Thus, for this type of smaller home, start-up costs appear to be minimal compared with those of purpose-built (or purpose-modified) facilities such as nursing homes or assisted-living settings (Kane, Wilson, and Clemmer 1993).

In contrast to information on fees from residents, board-and-care home operators had some difficulty in identifying dollar amounts for the ongoing expenses involved with providing housing and care. In part, this difficulty is logical, since few had purchased a home specifically to enable them to provide care (see chap. 2), so that their rent or mortgage was the same regardless of whether or not they had residents living with them. Many expenses, such as transportation, household expenses for food and cleaning products, and utilities were undoubtedly increased by the presence of the residents in the home. Yet operators had paid most of these same expenses routinely for their own households prior to the initiation of board-and-care services.

The extent to which many operators integrated the residents into their everyday lives meant that separating these additional expenses was often difficult for them. It appeared that in many homes the operators had not thought about the costs of operation in the way in which typical research studies would assess them. Our strategy, then, was to ask operators to gauge the *added* expenses in various categories involved in providing board-and-care services (i.e., how much *more* does transportation cost you a month because of your clients?). The data we present are therefore subject to methodological limitations. We anticipate that expenses were underestimated, while the fee amounts reported by operators were substantially more accurate.

Although a few operators kept strict and detailed accounts of expenses, others failed (or saw no reason) to separate family monies from resident fees in their everyday operation of the home. It was therefore difficult to gather accurate information on the ongoing expenses involved in small board-and-care homes. One interviewer described "some uneasy moments when discussion of expenses came up. They (a caregiver and her husband) provided the information and often corrected each other when estimates were too high or too low."

The high cost of more intensive, medically oriented care is driven by the salaries for personnel. Salaries for caregivers are a major component of the expense for care in most health care settings (Chen 1989; Conley 1989). In this light, it is important to point out that most of the small board-and-care home operators we studied did not pay themselves a "salary" in the regular sense. The financial benefit they received consisted of the profit, if any, generated by their care of residents. They contained costs of operation by providing services "voluntarily," sometimes with family support (Chen 1989). Baggett (1989) argues that it is in the service provision component of this work that many higher-cost residential care facilities make their profits. By taking more demanding (and thus higher-fee) residents, they move beyond basic room-and-board billing. Since, as we shall see, some members of our Baltimore sample made little or no profit once the expenses were paid, the operators would not have been able to afford to pay themselves a salary and continue to provide services. Whether this situation is oppressive toward the operators as workers is an issue that could easily be debated, since they often work long hours, seven days a week (Abel and Nelson 1990; Glazer 1990).

Regular Monthly Expenses

Prior research (Chen 1989; Mor, Gutkin, and Sherwood 1985) has examined expenses, finding that staffing and food account for two-thirds of the total expenses for the month. The percentage of total costs expended for food were higher in smaller homes, where staffing costs are modest, but food purchases cannot take advantage of economies of scale (Mor, Gutkin, and Sherwood 1985). Baltimore-area operators were asked to respond to a specific set of items reflecting areas of expense that could be expected to increase by virtue of the care provided for dependent adults in board-and-care. For each category, operators were asked how much they paid per month, whether the amount was increased by virtue of care for residents, and how much more the item cost monthly because of the residents. The results of the latter two items are summarized in table 2.

The percentage of operators reporting increased costs in particular areas ranged from very high (95.5 percent for groceries and household supplies and 93.1 percent for utilities) to quite low (10.0 percent for out-of-pocket health care costs and 7.4 percent for taxes). Most operators reported paying more for groceries, utilities, gifts/entertainment and recreation, staff or respite care providers, and transportation. Even when a significant percentage of operators said they were paying more for a particular item, the amounts were not consistently large.

The largest impact overall was, not surprisingly, from groceries and consumable household supplies. Almost all operators paid more in this

Table 2

Additional Routine Monthly Expenses Arising from Providing Care
in Baltimore Homes

Type of Expense	Percentage Reporting	Median ($)	Mean ($)	Range ($)
Groceries/supplies	95.5	300	421	0–2500
Utilities	93.1	100	113	0–375
Gifts/entertainment	78.8	20	57	0–1500
Staff or respite costs	73.7	100	335	0–5500
Transportation costs	69.8	38	84	0–600
Heat (if separate)	37.8	0	41	0–300
Home upkeep	34.2	0	65	0–1500
Telephone bill	18.2	0	12	0–400
Rent/mortgage	14.6	0	94	0–3010
Out-of-pocket health costs	10.0	0	12	0–200
Taxes	7.4	0	62	0–2400
Other	11.1	0	11	0–300

area, and the median per month spent for residents was $300, with figures
ranging up to $2,500 per month. Although most operators reported added
transportation costs and expenditures for gifts and entertainment, the
median dollar amounts spent in these areas were quite modest ($38 and
$20, respectively). Despite the relatively small dollar amounts, however,
these costs can amount to significant levels on an annual basis.

Overall, the median per-resident cost of operation was $491 per month
(1990 dollars). This figure was undoubtedly pulled downward by the reports of a few operators claiming that there were no expenses involved in
operating their homes and upward by the few operators claiming very
high expenses. The per-resident figure was, nonetheless, lower than
amounts in some prior studies, a result that may arise from differing methodologies and samples as well as variation in quality or types of services
available in the homes (see Chen 1989).

Extra Expenses

Aside from the routine monthly expenses involved in providing board-
and-care, operators told our interviewers that they often did additional
things for their residents, especially because many residents were on very
limited incomes. The operators also described unexpected expenses that
sometimes threatened the fragile financial balance of their homes. We
invited operators to tell us the various ways they spent their own money
on residents of the home and how much they spent in a typical month on

these "extras." Some of the categories offered by the operators overlap with the routine expenses mentioned above, but this question focused specifically on areas in which the operators would spend their money on clients. These responses, then, reflect the types of expenditures that go beyond the funds residents bring into the home for their maintenance. To understand the total picture of the expenses involved in home operation, these so-called extra expenses must be taken into account.

Operators were invited to tell whether they regularly or sometimes spent money on eight types of expenses that we had heard mentioned by operators during earlier interviews. They were also asked to list other kinds of extra expenses not included in our list and to summarize what these items cost them in a typical month. Holiday and birthday gifts were the most commonly mentioned types of extra expense coming from the operator's own funds (94.4 percent spent money on this item, 70.5 percent did so regularly). Nearly equal percentages of operators (68.2 percent [52.3 percent regularly] and 66.3 percent [24.7 percent regularly]) also spent their own funds on toiletries or clothing for residents. Over one-half of operators who answered said that they spent additional funds on over-the-counter medicines (58.0 percent) or transportation (53.0 percent) for residents. Fewer than half regularly expended funds for books and magazines, health products (such as adult diapers), or prescription medicines. Asked to estimate their total monthly expenditures from all of these extras, the

Table 3

Extra "Out-of-Pocket" Monthly Expenses to Operators in Baltimore Homes

	Percentage Reporting Expense	
Type of Expense	Occasionally	Regularly
Gifts (birthday/holiday)	23.9	70.5
Toiletries	15.9	52.3
Resident clothing	41.6	24.7
Over-the-counter medicines	29.8	28.2
Transportation	11.8	41.2
Books/magazines	17.0	26.1
Health products	14.9	20.7
Prescription medicines	5.7	5.7
Total spent on these extras:	Median, $60	
	Mean, $73	
	Range, $0–400	

median figure for all operators was $60, with a range from nothing to $400.

The most commonly reported (11.7 percent) expense that we had not listed was that for barber or hairdresser services. Other volunteered expenses included the purchases of cigarettes for residents, special gourmet foods or "treats," recreational activities, and other extras (4.9 percent each). According to these responses, most operators were called upon to spend money beyond what they regarded as "normal" expenditures in order to operate their board-and-care homes. For example, a Baltimore operator related an example of one of her clients who had skin problems requiring special care. The operator had difficulty getting the resident's husband to bring items like lotion, powder, or baby oil for this care. Since the husband only brought sample sizes, the operator would go out and buy the items herself, drawing the line at incontinence supplies that went beyond her budget. Another told of receiving $275 per month to care for a client. When a social worker asked how much she got as a clothing allowance, the operator replied that she received nothing. "The social worker asked, 'Well, how do you pay for his clothes?' 'My husband and I buy them for him,' I told her." Often these expenditures add up to significant amounts and cover an array of unmet needs (or choices by the operator) for the care of board-and-care clients.

Sometimes extra expenses can make all the difference. One operator told of facing a decision regarding whether to place a client with a growing problem of incontinence in a nursing home. "What can I do? We have replaced three mattresses since she moved in, seven pillows and three bedspreads. I've started to buy her sheets from Goodwill, because they are so expensive and, from all the washing and bleaching that I have to do to keep them clean, they ruin so easily. They won't reimburse me for the damaged goods." Another recounted how a young male client, who had moved in from living on the street "ran my telephone bill to $300 by calling that 'sex number.' I told him I could have *bought* him a woman for $300."

Overall Expenses of Operation

If we add up the dollar figures per month for the routine expenses and the "extras" spent by operators, we get an figure representing the operators' estimates of the ongoing costs of operation. The distribution on this expense measure showed a wide range across homes, from $0 (reported in seven homes) to $10,125 per month. The median value was a modest $545, but the mean ($961) was obviously pulled upward by the few high-expense homes ($N = 3$) above $5,000 per month. Since we did not go through financial records (assuming that there had been such records) or any formal accounting procedure to determine these expense figures, they are subject to the recall of operators. It would seem quite unlikely that an operator spent no additional money to care for one or more dependent adults in the home, nor is the $10,125 figure likely to be unbiased by omissions or exaggerations in various areas. The great majority of operators, however, gave us modest and plausible figures (42.8 percent fell between $300 and $1,000 per month).

Differences in monthly expenses by the operator's race were just barely significant, with median values of $495 for African American operators and $750 for white operators. As would be expected, expenses were substantially (and significantly) higher in larger homes (four to eight residents, median of $1,375, compared with $437 in homes with three or fewer residents). The modest difference in expenses between homes above or below the median fee (expenses were $446 for lower-fee and $620 for higher-fee homes) was not statistically significant, nor was the difference between homes participating in Project HOME (median, $510) and those not participating (median, $585). In all, given that African American operators tended to have smaller homes, these differences are reflections of closely aligned phenomena.

The expenses included in our figures do not include any salary or payment for the board-and-care home operator. Obviously those operators who were losing money would not be able to receive any income from their efforts, a source of potential problems for both those operators and their residents. Loss of just one resident could mean the difference between profit and loss. One operator recalled being forced to raise fees because she found herself routinely "dipping into my savings to make ends meet."

This absence of a salaried position also means that operators lack benefits and protections included in most jobs, such as workers compensation coverage, health insurance, and unemployment or pension benefits, including Social Security. Not only do they lack a reliable income, then, but they also lack the protections available to workers in most types of salaried health care employment. We also uncovered some apparent legal ambiguity regarding the status of the money paid to operators to provide care. According to the Project HOME program, the funds received by their operators are not income, and operators are not being paid for their time. Instead the funds are viewed as covering the costs of maintaining residents in the homes. Yet when one Project HOME operator tried to receive medical assistance for her family based on her income (excluding Project HOME revenue), she was declared ineligible because those fees *were* considered income by the Medical Assistance program. This operator was forced to take an additional job as a home health aide in order to have health insurance for herself and her two children. As another participating operator stated, "The money isn't supposed to be considered income, but how can you not think about it that way? When the client is gone and that money is not coming in, you have to make adjustments. I know I'm dreaming, but it would be nice if they would give us some type of supplement to help us keep our homes open while we are waiting for a new client. That would be nice."

Profitability

Economic Profit

A fundamental question for the continued viability of small board-and-care homes is whether they experience a profit (i.e., more income coming from providing board-and-care services than expenses arising from these services). Some prior research (Mor, Gutkin, and Sherwood 1985; Traxler 1983) has found homes operating at a monthly loss, with the deficit covered by other sources of income (Chen 1989). Chen (1989) found that higher fees did not automatically generate higher profits in a small sample of homes varying in size, because economies of scale enabled larger homes to control staffing costs. It should be emphasized that the homes we studied are private, ostensibly for-profit establishments (Dittmar et al. 1983; Stone and Newcomer 1985). Yet board-and-care does not fit neatly into this category because of the publicly funded nature of their services to many of their residents (see chap. 1; Newman 1989). Thus, the issue of profits and whether they actually serve as income to home operators is ambiguous.

To gain some insight into the prevalence and size of profits, we subtracted the rough measure of expenses available from our data from the more reliable information regarding income from fees. The resulting distribution of monthly profits ranged from −$1,016 to $6,005. This broad distribution is somewhat misleading, however, since most homes were far removed from the upper extreme. If the dollar range is divided into equal quarters, 34.7 percent (34 homes) are in the lowest segment (under $750), an additional 53 homes (54.1 percent) are in the second segment (under $2450), and only 11 homes occupy the top two-quarters of the dollar range of profits, with only 2 in the top quarter.

About 8 percent of homes for which we were able to calculate profitability ($N = 98$) reported a loss when comparing expenses with income on a monthly basis. The remainder showed some level of profit, with a median for all homes of $972 per month. As table 4 shows, the amount of profit varied somewhat across the types of homes compared, but many of the variations are smaller than expected.

Analyses of profits by the major categories of size of the home, the

Table 4
Profit Levels of Baltimore Homes, by Characteristics of Home Operator

Profit	All	Size		Race		Project HOME	
		1–3	4–8	Black	White	Yes	No
Per home							
Percentage with monthly loss	8.0	6.0	13.3	6.1	6.7	8.1	8.3
Median profit	$972	$949	$1,538	$933	$1,261	$1,216	$831
Lowest profit	–$1,016	–$1,016	–$369	–$950	–$1,016	–$950	–$1,016
Highest profit	$6,005	$3,724	$6,005	$3,724	$6,005	$4,173	$6,006
Per resident							
Percentage with monthly loss	7.1	6.0	13.3	6.1	6.7	8.1	8.3
Median profit	$491	$520	$254	$434	$539	$636	$322
Lowest profit	–$1,015	–$1,015	–$84	–$475	–$1,015	–$475	–$1,015
Highest profit	$1,862	$1,862	$835	$1,862	$1,075	$1,011	$1,075

Note: Profit is defined as the difference (positive or negative) between the home's income from providing care and the added routine and special expenses involved with providing care.

operator's race, and participation in Project HOME showed some interesting differences. Profits were significantly higher for white than for African American operators (medians, $1,261 vs. $933); and, perhaps not surprisingly, profits were significantly higher in homes with at least four residents compared to those with three or fewer (medians, $1,538 vs. $949). Also as anticipated, profits were significantly higher in homes with above average fees per resident than in those that were less expensive (medians, $1,296 vs. $784). Profits were not significantly different for homes with residents receiving subsidies from Project HOME, but the difference in profits was in favor of the participating homes. Larger homes were slightly more likely to face an operating loss, but having more residents created more of a cushion to enable payment of ongoing expenses.

Another way of examining profit is to discover the amount of profit per resident, reflecting, in essence, the payment received by each operator for the care given to that individual. As mentioned earlier, the median value for all residents was $491 per month across all homes (See table 4). Like the total profit to the home, profit per resident ranged from a negative value (−$1015) to a substantial positive figure ($1862), with few homes at the extreme of the distribution.

Per-resident profit varied in some different ways from the per-home profit. Specifically, the per-resident figures showed a lower median profit in larger homes than in smaller ones, with more of the larger homes having a monthly per-resident loss. Per-resident profits were similar to total profits, however, in that white operators still fared better than their African American counterparts, and Project HOME facilities reported nearly twice the per-resident profit each month that was reported for nonparticipating homes.

The profile of home profits looked quite different, however, when we included a fixed salary for the home operator as part of the expenses. We made two different estimations, reflected in figure 11. Using the basic income and expense information gathered from the operators, we added a hypothetical salary for the operator to the expense figure. In the first case, we added an operator salary of $10,000 per year to the expenses of the home. In the second, a salary of $25,000 per year was used. Since there is no established rate of pay for providing care of this type, often to multiple residents, these two benchmarks served as a modest and more generous level of remuneration to the board-and-care home operators for their services.

When the modest salary level was applied, the percentage of homes that experienced losses jumped from 8 percent to 40.8 percent. In this scenario, some homes lost up to $1,849 per month when this salary figure was included, and the highest monthly profit was reduced to $5,172. The

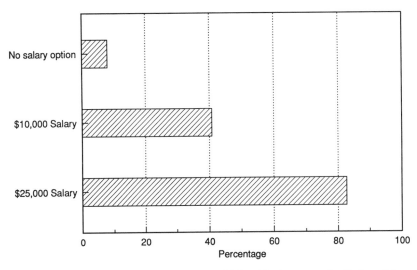

Fig. 11. Percentage of Baltimore Homes with Monthly Losses under Various Salary Assumptions

more generous salary assumption resulted in 82.7 percent of homes losing money on a monthly basis, with the largest loss reaching $3,099 per month and the profit of the most-advantaged home shrinking to $3,922. Clearly, the fact that many operators did not take a regular salary was critical to the continued "profit" of these homes.

Many homes could ill afford to provide their operators with the modest $10,000 per year salary without exceeding their monthly incomes, often by a considerable amount. The larger salary was even less practical, throwing between 50 and 86.7 percent of homes in the various groups (i.e., size, operator race, participation in Project HOME) into the monthly loss category. The current reimbursement system relies on the assumption that operators draw no salary or very low amounts from the provision of board-and-care services, especially in the homes providing care to those receiving only SSI or modest Social Security benefits to cover their needs.

From a critical point of view, the unreimbursed labor of the home operators, especially in the least profitable homes, could be interpreted as unfair. Since it is only by forgoing a modest wage that many homes remained profitable, the operation of small homes was predicated on this labor contribution by operators. The willingness of many operators to give care for an amount below minimum wage may be counterbalanced in their eyes by the autonomy afforded them in this type of caregiving as well as the interpersonal gratifications described in subsequent chapters. Overall, a wide range of profitability was encountered in the small board-and-care homes we studied in Baltimore.

Other "Profits" from Board-and-Care

The absence of a salary for the operators was, in some cases, partly counterbalanced by other noneconomic rewards or financial benefits that they received (see Chen 1989). We asked Baltimore operators, "What financial benefits (if any) do you get, other than the money, from caring for your clients?" In the open-ended response format, most operators could think of no such indirect, financial benefits.

Among those giving a response, however, 7.4 percent of operators said that operating a small board-and-care home either lowered their living costs or enabled them to earn more, so that money was not as tight. A smaller group (4.6 percent) responded either that they were able to afford a larger house than otherwise or that they could avoid child care costs by working at home. Smaller numbers (2.8 percent) reported being able to afford housing in a better neighborhood or being able to quit outside work (1.9 percent). A few operators also reported receiving lump-sum payments or funds from estates of their residents who had died. Although these indirect financial benefits were not major phenomena in our data, they should not be overlooked as important to the quality of life in recruiting or retaining operators for small homes.

Making Ends Meet: Other Sources of Income

It is important to point out that in contrast to purpose-built facilities with staff, small board-and-care homes received income from sources other than resident fees. In fact, without these other sources of income, homes operating at a loss or with low profits would be required to cease operation as board-and-care homes. Either the operators themselves or other members of their families in the household were employed, received pensions, or may have had other sources of income. The household economy did not, in all cases, rely upon the fees from board-and-care residents to make ends meet.

Reported levels of household income in the two study locations showed wide variations. Nearly half of Baltimore home operators (49.5 percent) reported household incomes under $25,000 (1989 dollars), and 72.5 percent reported levels below $40,000 from all sources (5.5 percent refused to respond to this question). Slightly more (58.3 percent) Cleveland operators reported household/family incomes under $25,000 (1985–86 dollars), and a similarly larger figure (81.3 percent) had family incomes under $40,000 (5.8 percent refused to respond). In general, the households were not wealthy, but often their incomes were derived from multiple sources, not simply board-and-care work. In fact, poorer operators (i.e., those with low fees or few clients) said that the earnings or income from other sources subsidized the needs of board-and-care residents in some cases. An example of how the other resources can make a difference appeared in an interviewer's notes on an operator whose "husband became a disabled veteran and was entitled to certain benefits. The sicker he got, the more support he received from the government (e.g., a van, a home, up to $4,000 per month). These extras allowed her to take in people who had nothing and provide for them. If she had not had these resources, she said she could not have supported them and cared for them in her home." Thus, we find that in many cases board-and-care operators were themselves financially marginal, a case of the moderately poor helping the very poor.

The first component of this other income was the earnings of the operator. About one in four Baltimore-area operators was employed outside the home. Perhaps surprisingly, most of these jobs were not in health care and ranged from teaching to waitressing. Operators reported that they worked a wide range of hours (three to forty hours per week; median, twenty), and most (68.8 percent) worked daytime hours. While this may seem problematic (i.e., leaving residents without the care and assistance they need), the use of day programs enabled operators to continue employment, at least on a part-time basis, while caring for residents.

Although we did not specifically inquire about other sources of income, the presence of spouses, many of whom were employed, and the likelihood of other sources of income (e.g., pensions, disability benefits, income from providing respite care) may mean that the income from board-and-care was less central to the household. In cases where operators' costs exceeded their income from fees, these other sources of income enabled the continued provision of services to the dependent adults housed in the board-and-care home.

Money Management

Money management issues that faced the homes involved both the operators and their running of the home and the residents themselves. Concerns have been raised regarding the ethical dilemmas that arise when operators are involved in managing financial affairs for severely impaired and dependent individuals. We address first the involvement of operators and others in the money management of residents and then turn to financial management of the board-and-care home by the operator and others.

The Residents' Money

Money management by and for the residents of board-and-care homes may occur outside the home and beyond the involvement of the operator. In other instances, however, the operators of homes assist their residents with managing their money. Although, as was shown in chapter 2, many home operators offered business and financial management as a service to residents (63.7 percent by Baltimore operators), fewer residents actually used such assistance.

In Cleveland, 24.5 percent of operators reported that they were handling the finances for one or more residents in their homes at the time of the interview. Among the cognitively intact Cleveland residents interviewed, about half (53.2 percent) reported that they needed help managing money. While over half of those needing help reported getting it, the help was five times more likely to come from a family member than from the operator of the home or other staff there. The operator or staff were much more likely to assist African American residents (23.5 percent vs. 5.4 percent), and twice as many white residents (61.1 percent vs. 31.4 percent) received help from their families, a statistically significant difference. Families were also relied upon more by residents in higher-fee homes, with operators significantly less likely to manage finances for residents in those homes. We speculate that the levels of operator assistance with finances would be higher among residents with significant cognitive impairment, who were unable to answer the interview in Cleveland. In many cases, then, operators were not involved in the money management of their residents, but they were more likely to assist those who were the most vulnerable or impaired.

Methods of Payment

A related issue of financial control involved the means by which operators were paid for their services. Some policymakers have raised concerns about making home operators, who exert considerable control over the lives of their more dependent clients, representative payees. When operators are representative payees, they receive, and have the power to cash, checks for benefits to their residents, opening the possibility for fraud or abuse. Many programs pay the care providers directly, rather than having funds pass through the hands of dependent adults, many of whom would be unable to manage the money because of their physical or mental disabilities (CSSP 1988; Dobkin 1989).

Operators in Baltimore were asked (for up to four residents at the second interview) how each one paid for housing and services. Multiple responses for any given resident were possible. Figure 12 outlines the percentages of Baltimore operators who reported that they were receiving fees for resident care through each of five specific methods. Operators were counted in these percentages if they reported using each means of payment for at least one of their current residents. About one-third of the operators reported that they were representative payees, receiving checks directly for their dependent residents. Being a representative payee was significantly more likely among African American operators in this sample.

Being paid by the family was the second most common method and was significantly more prevalent in larger homes (53.3 percent vs. 22.7 percent) and those with white operators. Clients paid the operator directly in fewer than one in four homes, but this was more common in homes charging below average fees (34.5 percent vs. 10.4 in higher-fee homes). Operators of nearly one home in five reported that at least some clients' fees were paid directly by a social service program or agency, while in 17.5 percent of homes at least one client signed over her or his check to the operator. This diversity of means by which operators receive their money included more reliable (representative payee, program/agency payment) methods and methods subject to the control of or abuse by the client or client's family (client pays directly, family pays or client signs over check). Whether this control by the residents or their families resulted in more autonomy or

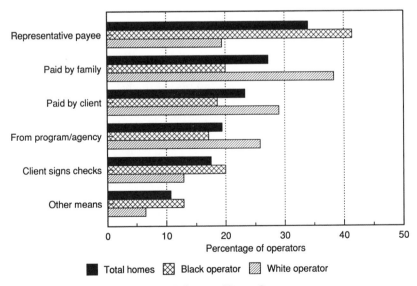

Fig. 12. Methods of Payment to Baltimore Home Operators

simply more risk of nonpayment or late payment to the operator was unclear. Anecdotally, some operators reported that payments were sometimes late or that they had trouble with being paid by certain residents (or their families), who were often asked to move because of this problem.

How Operators Manage Their Finances

Given the small scale of these board-and-care homes, financial management does not raise the same level of concern as it would in a larger, more formal organization. Yet operators must manage their monthly budgets, pay taxes, and sometimes meet a payroll. Questions in the second interview of Baltimore home operators addressed concerns related to money management by home operators. Other questions (described later in the chapter) examined their attitudes toward financial issues, including money management, in further detail.

Few of the operators (3.9 percent) reported relying on someone else exclusively for the handling of "day-to-day finances (paying bills, keeping records)." Most operators reported doing these tasks themselves (59.2 percent) or combining their efforts with those of another person (23.3 percent). Although operators in larger homes were somewhat less likely to be self-reliant in money management, there were no significant differences in their responses to this question by home size, operator race, or the average fee paid in the home.

With those who had partial or complete help in handling finances, we inquired about who provided that help. Nearly half of those responding (46.7 percent) received help from one of their family members, fewer from a tax preparer (23.3 percent), accountant (13.3 percent), or lawyer (6.7 percent). A few (10.0 percent) reported help from a combination of individuals. Most of those receiving help paid for the financial management services they received (56.7 percent). While virtually all of the financial professionals were paid, very few of the family helpers were reported to be receiving payment for their assistance. Yet few operators reported that their helpers did all or even most of the financial management tasks (23.3 percent). In most cases, despite having help, the operators did most of the ongoing money management in the households themselves.

The relative informality of the business side of small board-and-care homes was reinforced by the findings on record keeping. We asked home operators whether they kept written records on nine types of information pertaining to their residents and home operation. As the findings in figure 13 show, record keeping was variable and significantly less extensive than that found in more formal health care organizations (Diamond 1990). For example, Dittmar and associates (1983) found that nearly all operators in

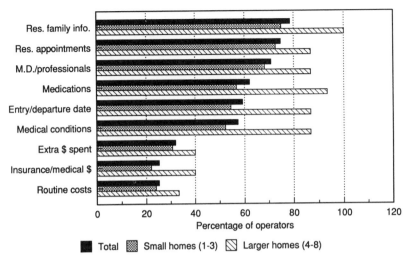

Fig. 13. Percentage of Baltimore Operators Keeping Written Records of Various Kinds

the larger board-and-care homes they studied kept records, including signed admission agreements (78.1 percent), names of physicians (97.0 percent), and accident reports (86.7 percent).

Nearly four out of five Baltimore homes kept written records of residents' families, a type of information kept by all of the larger homes. Fewer homes kept information on resident medical and other appointments (74.8 percent), records of physician and other medical professionals working with residents (70.9 percent), and on clients' medications (62.1 percent).

Interestingly for our purposes here, the three lowest rates of record keeping had to do with financial issues. Between one-third and one-quarter of homes kept records of extra money spent on residents, insurance or medical expenses of residents, or everyday costs of operation. Although limited record keeping with regard to resident medical expenses may be logical, since operators seem to be largely uninvolved in payment for these services, the other two forms of record keeping would appear to be required in most instances where a small business was being operated. The fact that few operators kept such records reflected their attitudes toward the financial side of home operation (discussed in a later section of this chapter).

Homes were more similar than dissimilar in terms of record keeping. In general, the larger homes were more likely to keep records than those housing three or fewer residents, nearly half of whites (48.4 percent vs. 14.3 percent of African Americans) operating homes kept records of everyday costs of operation, and high-fee homes acted somewhat more "medical" in that higher percentages kept medication records (73.5 percent versus 51.0 percent in lower-fee homes) and charts of medical conditions of residents (67.3 percent vs. 46.9 percent).

In spite of an expectation that those operators participating in Project HOME might be required to keep more detailed records, their level of record keeping was mostly similar to that of other, nonparticipating operators. On only one item, the everyday costs of home operation, were they significantly more likely to keep records than their peers. Overall, record keeping in small board-and-care homes was limited to the most essential information. Operators apparently did not perceive the need to maintain the extensive records that characterize medically oriented facilities, nor did regulations require extensive charting from them in most cases.

Attitudes toward Money by Operators

One striking issue that appeared from our repeated visits with operators of small board-and-care homes was their attitude toward money and its importance. Although there was variation among operators in these attitudes, many of them disavowed financial gain as the major motivating factor in providing board-and-care services. Among the operators from the Cleveland area, for example, when asked "How did you start taking people into your home?" relatively few (16.6 percent) mentioned economic necessity, and 15.8 percent wanted to "make a business." When asked about their "major reasons for continuing to do this?" more operators mentioned financial necessity (28 percent), but fewer mentioned interest in creating a business (4.3 percent).

More operators focused on providing service as their motivation for continuing to work in the board-and-care field. One Baltimore operator adamantly declared to the interviewer at each visit that her goal was to keep elderly people out of nursing homes. She didn't consider what she did to be running a business, but saw herself as providing people with a home and someone to care for them when they need it. Her fees were negotiable, and she took clients on SSI. One major concern she voiced was getting clients covered by medical assistance for their medical expenses. "I've had lots of people tell me that I have quite a business, but I *don't* do this for the money. Money *is* a concern though. It has to be. How else am I going to run this home?"

A series of items included in the first and second interviews with Baltimore-area operators involved their attitudes toward and problems with money. Some of these items were mixed in with other questions measuring burden (see chap. 4) and motivation to avoid response-set bias. Responses ranged from "strongly agree" to "strongly disagree," and results in table 5 show the percentage of operators who "agreed" or "strongly agreed" with each of the statements. Most operators agreed that they didn't earn enough money for their work and that they faced a lot of unexpected costs, with both of these attitudes being fairly invariant across home size, race of the operator, and fee levels in the homes. Fewer operators reported worrying about the costs of running the home (31.9 percent), although more white operators and those in homes with four to eight residents agreed with this statement. Similarly, fewer than one in five operators thought managing money was too much trouble, an attitude that was especially rare among operators of higher-fee homes (11.1 percent).

Ambivalence in their feelings about finances were apparent in these attitudinal responses. Most operators agreed with both a statement of preference to continue operating the home "even if I could make more money doing something else" (85.7) and one stating that they take care of people in their homes more "because I want to help, rather than for money" (86.8 percent). Yet nearly as many acknowledged that "the income I receive is very important to allow me to continue to offer this service" (84.6 percent), and a smaller, but substantial, minority (39.6 percent) admitted that "it would be hard for me to stop running a board-and-care home now, because I rely on that income to help support me." Interestingly, operators not participating in Project HOME were slightly more likely to agree with this last statement, although the difference did not quite reach statistical significance. Despite receiving generally higher fees, however, the Project HOME operators did not demonstrate attitudes that differed significantly from those of other operators on any of these items.

One married couple operating a successful home told our interviewer that they had started the home as a way to help people, but had become financially dependent and could not easily stop now. The husband said, "It would be like changing careers." Another stated strongly that she did not do what she does for the money. Financially stable because of her husband's military disability status, she stated, "You must do this for *more* than the money! You have to like people, know how to listen to them." Another operator responded, when asked to reflect about whether she worried about the costs of running her home, "I just do it. I don't worry about it. It isn't enough [money] and that's a fact, but I got to do it."

Failure of the financing mechanisms supporting medical care to meet the needs of patients sometimes necessitates turning to the board-and-care industry for assistance. Case notes revealed a story that is probably not

Table 5

Baltimore Operator Reactions to Financial Aspects of Providing Care

| | Percentage Who "Agree" or "Strongly Agree" | | | | | | |
| | Size of Home | | Race of Operator | | Resident Fees | |
Statement	All	1–3	4–8	Black	White	Low	High
I don't earn enough money for the amount of work that I do.	56.0	55.3	51.1	59.0	50.0	62.8	51.1
I worry a lot about the costs of running this home.	31.9	26.3	60.0*	24.6	46.4*	32.6	31.1
There are a lot of unexpected costs in running a . . . home.	52.7	51.3	60.0	50.8	53.6	53.5	51.1
(T)he money I get from caring for my clients is enough to cover (things) they need.	44.0	46.1	33.3	39.3	57.1	39.5	46.7
Managing money and doing taxes is too much trouble for someone running a home like this.	19.8	19.7	20.0	18.0	21.4	27.9	11.1*
The income I receive is very important to allow me to continue to offer this service.	84.6	84.2	86.7	82.0	89.3	83.7	84.4
I would prefer to continue operating this home, even if I could make more money doing something else.	85.7	85.5	86.7	85.2	85.7	88.4	82.2
I take care of people in my home more because I want to help, rather than for money.	86.8	88.2	80.0	93.4	71.4*	88.4	84.4
It would be hard for me to stop running (a home) now, because I rely on that income to help support me.	39.6	40.8	33.3	36.1	46.4	44.2	33.3
I think of what I am doing mostly as running a business.	19.8	19.7	20.0	19.7	21.4	20.9	20.0

*Differences between groups statistically significant at $p < .05$.

unusual. A physician called one of the operators in our Baltimore sample about keeping an elderly female whose Medicare and Blue Cross coverage had run out while she was in the hospital. The client needed total care. The physician asked if the operator could keep the client until readmission to the hospital was possible. The operator kept the client for sixty days and received no reimbursement for this care. When asked if she though that the situation was unfair, she adamantly stated, "Absolutely not. I don't do this for money. I'm here to help these people as much and whenever I can."

Clearly the operators' recognition of the financial aspects of board-and-care was somewhat grudging. They acknowledged its importance in providing the means to continue their work, but, in their own minds, they minimized the importance of money in comparison to the service they were providing to others and to the interpersonal aspects of giving care. A male operator, according to interviewer field notes, "admitted that economic rewards were a primary benefit (of running his home). The business enabled him to get out of debt after purchasing this home. But he also stated, 'If Project HOME stopped its program tomorrow, I would keep these people with me even though their only income would be SSI.'"

A final question of interest, given this apparent ambivalence among the operators, asked whether they "think of what [they are] doing mostly as running a business." Only one in five operators agreed with this statement; most of those responding strongly disagreed. As one operator reported, "When someone does this as a business, they expect money for themselves. I get their money and buy them everything they need." There was no variation in this attitude by the race of the operator, size of the home, or the fee level currently being charged. Apparently operators recognize the business side of board-and-care but prefer not to emphasize it in their own thinking about what they do.

When the operators in Baltimore were given the opportunity to elaborate on why their board-and-care homes were or were not like a business, a variety of responses appeared. Among the answers (up to two answers per operator were coded) to the open-ended question, 37.4 percent of operators mentioned that the homes were "like family," 24.4 percent emphasized the "loving and giving" nature of their care homes, 15.4 percent said that their homes lacked the traits of a business, such as having staff and a payroll, while others (13.2 percent) emphasized the service nature of the work they did. According to one operator, "It's a *care* home—I would quit if it became a business."

Other operators (31.9 percent) mentioned that the home was, in fact, a business, but few other justifications were provided for this position. Curiously, a few operators who said that board-and-care *was* a business also saw it as "like family" or emphasized the service work and personal care aspects (see chap. 6). It seems as though the operators saw an apparent contradiction in the business side of board-and-care and the very personal relationships of the service work.

Another view of the attitudes toward money was provided by a question asked in the fourth interview in Baltimore. Once we had established that many operators did not feel that they were being paid enough for their work, we asked them, "What do you think would be a fair monthly fee for the average client you have had here in the past year?" Answers, which tended to come in even amounts, ranged from $200 to $3,000 per month, with a median of $1,025 (mean, $1,529). The means were skewed upward by the two operators who claimed that $3,000 was their "fair fee." Although figures differed by the number of residents in the home (medians: $1,000 for operators of homes with one to three residents, $1,500 for those with four to eight residents), the difference was not statistically significant by analysis of variance. Nor were the very small differences by operator's race (medians: $1,000 for African American operators, $1,050 for white operators) statistically significant.

The fee level considered "fair" differed as a function of the fees currently being charged in the homes. Operators currently charging higher-than-average fees expected more as a fair fee (median, $1,500; mean, $2,103) than did those currently receiving sums in the lower half of the distribution of current fees (median, $1,000; mean, $1,003). It is not surprising that the higher-fee operators felt that their current price structure was justified and believed that their work warranted greater remuneration. Inclusion of the two operators desiring $3,000 per month in this group was sufficient to create this significant difference.

Clearly, the operators recognized the essential role of money and "business aspects" in their small board-and-care homes. Their attitudes toward the financial side were mixed with feelings that they should not be overly concerned about economic matters, but instead should focus their energies on the care that they provide to residents. Most operators, except the few claiming fees at the lowest end as "fair," expressed the sentiment that they were underpaid to some degree. Most were, nonetheless, continuing to provide board-and-care services in their homes.

Elite Homes: Some Important Contrasts

Although the bulk of the homes studied in both locations were modest in terms of their fees, services, and profitability, we identified four homes in Baltimore that might be considered elite in a financial sense. Home sizes ranged from two residents to our sample's maximum of eight, and as mentioned earlier, none participated in Project HOME. Geographical sites ranged from urban to rural. These elite homes tended to offer all of the services described in chapter 2 (see fig. 7) except assistance for clients in managing finances and business affairs, which was available in only two of these four homes.

All of the residents in these select homes were over age sixty-five, white, and without a history of hospitalization for mental illness. They also differed from the overall resident population in that most (68 percent) had children, and more than was the case for typical residents, they received income from Social Security Retirement and other pensions.

These four homes charged fees that sometimes varied across residents, but whose median amount was at or above $1,500 per month per resident, with the lowest individual fee reported at $1,283 per month. Both operators claiming $3,000 as their "fair fee" amount were in this small group of elite homes. Total income to the home from providing board-and-care services ranged from $3,724 to $16,006 per month. These operators also tended to claim among the highest amounts for monthly expenses, including the one reporting $10,125 per month in operating costs. This operator included an extensive paid staff in her home (housekeeper, chef, nursing assistants, craft worker, and musician), accounting for much of this cost. She offered classes to residents to avoid boredom (crafts, cooking, and music) and reported that no one from her family, the neighborhood (friends, neighbors), or the residents' families assisted in her work in any way. Another operator in this elite group, in contrast, relied almost entirely on relatives living within the home for backup, maintenance, and personal care of residents.

Since one of these homes dropped out of the study following the first interview, we lack information on her operating expenses. Interestingly, however, among the remaining three "elite" operators, one claimed no costs involved in running her home (with two residents). The remaining two had more-expected figures of $6,410 and $8,030 per month in routine expenses. Profits (assuming no salary for the operators) ranged from one negative value (−$335 per month) to $6,005, with all but the one negative value above $3,700 per month. The one negative value resulted from the operator's report of high expenses for a small number of residents.

Perhaps surprisingly, home operators in this elite group were diverse in some ways. Two were white, one Asian American, and one African American. One of the four was employed outside the home. Their household incomes were all above $30,000 per year, and all of these elite operators housed exclusively older persons, avoiding the younger, mentally ill population. Not surprisingly, all of these homes provided private rooms for their residents.

Despite the potential for greater relevance of money in these homes, these operators mirrored many of the attitudes of other operators (e.g., preferring board-and-care to other work for more money and disagreeing that what they do is primarily "running a business"). Despite higher levels of amenities and often higher profits, the operators of financially elite homes still disavowed the importance of money in their interviews with us.

Economic Marginality: Implications of Being in the Irregular Economy

As these data have demonstrated, small board-and-care homes operated on a financially marginal basis, often able to continue operation only because the operators took less than a market wage for their work. There is, however, another sense in which the economic aspects of small board-and-care homes, specifically those that were unregulated and unconnected to funding programs, demonstrated marginality—through their participation in the "irregular economy" (Ferman 1990).

Ferman describes the irregular economy as activity that is not recorded or monitored in the larger economy but in which money changes hands for goods or services (1990). This segment of economic activity is not counted in the overall productivity of the country or of those who participate in it. Among the key elements describing the irregular economy are small size, with one person typically acting as an entrepreneur; low levels of investment of time or money to initiate the enterprise; face-to-face negotiation of transactions between producer and consumer, idiosyncratic and particularistic price setting, often shaped by personal relationships between producer and consumer; and an intermediate level of skill required for the production of the good or service (Ferman 1990).

Finally, Ferman suggests that many of the services of the irregular economy are secured without fee by most individuals, usually from their informal networks of family and friends. "The irregular economy was generally utilized for services that most people secure without monetary payment and that are usually not provided by regular firms and businesses. The irregular sector seems to function as an alternative service provider in instances where the household is unable to perform the service or unable to have it done without payment. In this sense it fills an intermediate position between the regular market economy and do-it-yourself activities" (Ferman 1990, 124). In other words, Ferman recognized the marginality of irregular economy endeavors, such as board-and-care homes.

The parallels from this description of the irregular economy with the characteristics we have seen in the economic realm of small board-and-care homes are striking. Most homes are small, with essentially one person operating the establishment; little capital is invested to get the home into operation; fees are set in idiosyncratic ways, often taking the characteristics of the particular resident into consideration; exchange of fees, aside from those involved in programs, often takes place directly between the operator and the resident and family; and, as we will see in later chapters, the level of skill involved in providing care to typical residents is intermediate. Further description in a later chapter on residents will clarify the lack of close kin that warrants service provision outside the usual kin-caregiving channels.

In this view, small board-and-care homes, as part of the irregular economy, are filling an important gap for individuals with intermediate levels of impairment who lack close familial ties or the financial resources to buy necessary services. The do-it-yourself alternative of family caregiving works for most people requiring this level of assistance, but society lacks backup systems for individuals without those key familial supports. In this manner, small board-and-care homes, as an irregular economy adaptation to an unmet need, fill a gap between informal and formal groups, home and institution, that would otherwise leave many individuals displaced or with inappropriate types of care.

Although the irregular economy may provide necessary supports in certain areas and opportunities for entrepreneurship, there are some risks associated with participation in the irregular economy and its marginal position in the larger economy. Enterprises in the irregular economy may lack the legitimacy to gain resources from formal institutional sources (such as bank loans for home improvements or Medicaid reimbursement); the irregular economy may have problems with quality control (problems described in chap. 1); work opportunities are unpredictable (operators may have difficulty locating or retaining desirable residents); and unstructured prices and face-to-face dealings may mean difficulty in collecting fees for services (see also Enarson 1990). Workers in the irregular economy are not accorded the protections and benefits (e.g., pensions, workers compensation) of those employed in the regular sector (Ferman 1990). The unanswered question of why, given these difficulties, workers continue in the irregular economy may be partly answered by understanding the noneconomic motivations espoused by operators (see chap. 4).

In part, the status of operators as workers in the irregular economy may have to do with simple issues of supply and demand. When providers are giving good-quality service for a reasonable fee and there is high demand, they undoubtedly experience a high level of autonomy in their working environment. When there is an ample supply of spaces for those desiring care and when reputations are unestablished or questionable, those seeking services probably have somewhat more power in bargaining for services. If regulations drive some board-and-care homes underground (see Applebaum and Ritchie 1992), it might significantly enhance the bargaining power of those who employ the operators, residents and their kin, in negotiating for fees and services. Since a failure to comply with the demands of a customer could result in disclosure to authorities of the nonregulated caregiving environment, the balance of power in the relationship is shifted away from the operator (Enarson 1990).

One issue implicit in the discussions of introducing more regulation on small board-and-care homes is that this action would also move them from the irregular into the regular economy, with all of the formalization and bureaucratization that implies. Although the difficulties of marginality in the irregular economy would be largely removed, they would be replaced with a substantially different set of problems and issues for the operators. For example, regularity of payment from agency sources would be balanced by an increase in requirements for record keeping and attendance at training meetings. The nature of the work and the operator's autonomy within it would be changed dramatically by this action.

A real question remains as to whether a more regulated board-and-care system would be as able to meet the needs of the variety of individuals now being housed, especially the poor (Ehrlich 1986). Generally, with regulation comes an increase in costs, which may move the currently affordable board-and-care homes beyond the cost of poorer individuals, unless substantial subsidies are made available. The irregular economy can "flex" to meet many needs that emerge, with part-time or intermittent work, whereas the regular economy tends to be more constrained in dealing with unexpected or intermittent demands (Ferman 1990; Sussman 1978).

□ THE MARGINALITY of small board-and-care homes with regard to economic and financial issues is seen in both objective and subjective realms. In the objective area, we have already seen that the homes were often only breaking even or generating little profit, while a few appeared to be losing money when income and expenses were compared. The apparent willingness of operators to provide shelter and services to their clientele without profit or earnings for themselves gives testimony to the marginality of small board-and-care homes as businesses. Some operators continued to provide services (and others claimed they would) for residents who were temporarily unable to pay the usual fees. Thus, it appears that the operators defined the relationships with some clients as reaching beyond the fee-for-service model.

Turning to the subjective dimension, we also saw evidence that the small board-and-care home did not necessarily fit the operational model for a service business. Transferring financial management thinking from other care settings to small board-and-care homes met with only limited success. Generally, operation of a business or service requires income, provided as fees for goods and services from clientele. These funds are then budgeted to pay the necessary expenses of operation (facility, staff, food, etc.). Some of the homes we studied, especially larger ones, met this model fairly well, including structuring a salary for the home operator as part of the ongoing budget. Other operators used a very different model or approach to finances. They took income from all sources (resident fees, earnings, pensions, or other income from the operator and her coresident kin) and pooled it. From this pool of money, necessities were purchased and the mortgage was paid. Often the operators received no formal salary, and sometimes they took money from their pockets to provide extras for the residents. These two ends of a continuum demonstrate ways in which operators appear to handle the financial aspects of home operation. There were also those in between these two extremes who kept money separate in some instances but not in others. These varying approaches made it difficult for us to gain comparable information from the operators using diverse styles. Some operators had detailed, formal records of income and expenditures, while others simply made their expenses and income work out on a week-by-week basis, without advanced planning.

Financial issues are highly related to policy concerns and to the various programs and mandates that provide funding for the clients in many of the homes we studied. As Dittmar reflected (1989, 2), it has become clear that "the board and care industry was a private sector response to an existing need, that there was little regulation, and that the federal government was funding through SSI, a system of care over which it had little control." Often there was a lack of coordination between agencies and organizations, resulting in problems for the operators. For example, one elderly client, receiving Social Security ($337) and a small ($29) SSI check learned that she was due a small pension ($43 per month). This pension check had been sent to the client's previous address (and apparently cashed by relatives living there, reportedly to pay for an insurance policy of which neither the client nor the operator was previously aware). This additional $43 made the client ineligible for SSI and medical assistance. The operator asked, "What are we going to do? She can't afford her medicine and that little Social Security check barely covers other things she needs . . . I don't think she's nursing home material. What are they going to do with her if I don't keep her? . . . I *can't* afford to pay for her medicine."

These financial dilemmas and the marginality of the home operators are further detailed in chapter 4, which takes an in-depth look at the home operators and their concerns.

4 □ Operators of the Homes

□ OPERATORS SERVE as the linchpin for all activities in the board-and-care home and are thus central to a variety of issues regarding the quality of care, the provision of services, and the maintenance of a motivated work force (Newman 1989; Rubinstein 1995). From the perspective of some policymakers, operators are a resource to be cultivated to provide essential services in the community (Baggett 1989). The need to motivate and to maintain a supply of low-cost alternatives for care of the burgeoning population of dependent adults is, however, balanced by concerns over the potential for fraud and abuse should the providers prove incompetent (Hawes et al. 1993; Newman 1989). Policymakers and program administrators share with the public concerns about protecting the rights and safety of the dependent adults placed in board-and-care homes, reacting most often to the horror stories presented in the media and to local notorious operators who flaunt the laws and regulations.

Since the quality of care turns on the operator's abilities, issues such as training are often viewed as the key to enhancing the quality of board-and-care services (Dittmar and Smith 1983). Yet the work of operators can be viewed in a larger framework of women acting as caregivers. Both within the family and in more formally organized, paid settings, women are preponderant as the "hands-on" providers of services to dependent populations, often under the direction and management of men when in formal organizations (Abel and Nelson 1990). Expectations that women are appropriate to serve in these typically unappreciated and underpaid positions have led to charges that caregiving work is oppressive, limiting women's options in employment or in the home to the unchosen, boring, repetitive, instrumental tasks of maintaining society's dependent populations (i.e., children, the elderly, and the disabled). In this view, caregiving is a duty for women (Reverby 1990), rather than a choice.

An alternative view is that caregiving is a special skill of women, highlighting their nurturant sides for the betterment of society (Abel and Nelson 1990). In this view, women bring special value orientations and skill to the provision of care that enhances their success and satisfaction. For example, nurses, predominantly female, have adopted altruism as a fundamental value of their work, as well as being key to their nurturing roles as women in their families (Reverby 1990).

In essence, the board-and-care operators can be seen as a part of this tradition of caregiving, regardless of the ideological interpretation attached to it. Board-and-care home operators fall into a category of "unaffiliated providers," described by Abel and Nelson (1990). These unaffiliated providers, including home day care workers and midwives, are paid for their work but offer care in informal settings, such as the home. Abel and Nelson (1990) question whether unaffiliated caregivers are in control of their own working situations, since they often provide care in isolated settings. Having to negotiate directly for and collect their own fees, as well as potentially losing their clients unexpectedly, puts them in a disadvantaged position, also described as characteristic of the irregular economy (Ferman 1990). Abel and Nelson point out that the unaffiliated workers typically do not have a strictly defined set of tasks in their work and that they escape bureaucratic structures common to similar jobs in formal organizations (1990).

The role of the small home operator parallels those of several other fields that also fall under the heading of "unaffiliated provider." In each of these cases, the occupant of the job is faced with structural ambiguities that bridge the family and more formal organizations (i.e., they are socially marginal). The closest role is that found in the contemporary United Kingdom of warden of a sheltered care facility for elderly people (Butler, Oldman, and Greve 1983). The female-dominated job of warden provides a variety of services, from personal care and meals to general cleaning of common areas. She is also "on call" around the clock for emergencies through an alarm system and seldom gets time off from her duties, unless she arranges for someone to provide relief.

The warden was thought of (and is still by many) as the "good neighbor" who provides a natural, nonprofessional response to the dependency of tenants in the sheltered housing complex (Butler, Oldman, and Greve 1983). She undertakes any and all duties on an as-needed basis, a situation that can be problematic if a number of tenants significantly increase their levels of dependence. Wardens also often have husbands and children living with them, who may or may not assist in meeting the needs of the residents.

Parallels also appear with the preprofessional days of nursing, when care by nurses occurred in the home (Reverby 1990). Older widows or spinsters could "profess to" nursing in the marketplace and be hired by families to care for their sick, on the basis of experience with caring for a spouse or parent during illness. Being women was virtually their only qualification, and roles involved nonmedical care such as feeding, bathing, dressing, and transferring the patient.

According to research (Enarson 1990; Nelson 1990), day-care providers, another group of unaffiliated caregivers, align themselves with the role of mothering, rather than the more professional role of teaching, in their work. This orientation toward mothering creates dilemmas for the day-care workers, since they cannot exercise the rights and duties of parents. Instead, like operators of small board-and-care homes, they charge fees for providing care that they offer in their own homes. Therefore, limits must be placed around the emotional and social bonds that develop in the course of ongoing, daily contact in the home (Nelson 1990). Also like board-and-care operators, day-care providers can, to some degree, choose the number and type of children for whom they will provide services. They are free to reject a particular child or to consider the mix of ages and personalities in making selection decisions (Nelson 1990). But they may be compelled by economic pressures to accept children they dislike or feel ill-prepared to manage (Enarson 1990).

Nelson identifies "detached attachment," an unofficial and often unrecognized boundary marking the providers' need to protect themselves emotionally from the probable eventual loss of children in their care through maturation, relocation, or other causes (1990). Day-care providers attempt to distinguish between the emotional bonds of parenting and the more reserved emotional links they forge with children in day-care, also enabling them to reconcile charging fees for the "mothering" that they provide free to their own offspring.

As with other unaffiliated providers, operators of small board-and-care homes are workers in the "irregular economy." Their efforts exemplify being caught between professional and lay caregiving, between the formal long-term-care institutions and family care, and between the regulated medical world and the unregulated voluntary help provided to frail and dependent adults, including elderly people (Abel and Nelson 1990; Morgan, Eckert, and Lyon 1993).

The continued existence of small board-and-care homes is predicated on the availability and willingness of a cadre of workers, predominantly women, to perform this work and take dependent adults into their homes. This chapter profiles the board-and-care home operators in our two samples, describes the degree to which their work places them under a burden akin to that of families providing care, and describes how the operators construct and operate within a culture that defines the marginal relationships they hold with their resident clients.

Who are the Operators of Small Board-and-Care Homes?

As described above, the operators of small board-and-care homes demonstrate many characteristics similar to those of women who serve as caregivers in other paraprofessional settings. Examination of their demo-graphic traits, as well as their prior backgrounds, shows them to parallel the usual profile of those involved in caregiving work (Bartoldus, Gillery, and Sturges 1989; Braun, Horwitz, and Kaku 1988; Burgio and Burgio 1990; Feldman 1990; Kaye 1986; Sherman and Newman 1988). Their traits also identify them as part of "the 'underclass' of workers," on the basis of both demographic characteristics and the limited nature of their prior employ-ment (Applebaum and Phillips 1990, 448; Tellis-Nayak and Tellis-Nayak 1989).

Profile of Home Operators

The samples of operators from the Cleveland and Baltimore studies are profiled in table 6. In many ways the two samples are similar to each other and to findings of prior research on board-and-care homes (Sherman and Newman 1988). First, both samples had average ages in the fifties, with a wide range of ages represented (from the twenties to the seventies). Al-though the Baltimore operators had a higher average age, there were also other age differences among groups of operators. In Cleveland there were significant differences by home size and race, such that white operators and those with larger homes were younger than other operators. In both cities fees made a significant difference, in that younger operators tended to fall into the category of homes charging higher fees.

The ages reported here for operators are somewhat higher than those found in some other studies (e.g., Dittmar et al. 1983; Mor, Sherwood, and Gutkin 1986) and may represent a cause for some concern. The concentra-tion of operators of older ages raises two possibilities. One is that work in a small board-and-care home is an activity that providers come to in their later years, after trying other employment options. A second possibility is that the small board-and-care home industry is dying out, as reflected by the aging pool of operators (Dittmar 1989). It is unclear from our data whether either of these hypotheses is correct, but the aging of the operator pool, if it is occurring, raises important questions about the future of small board-and-care homes as an alternative for dependent adults.

One substantial difference between our two samples was that most operators in the Baltimore area were African Americans, compared with 29.5 percent of the operators in Cleveland (see table 6). To some extent this represents the difference in the racial makeup of the two metropolitan areas and the fact that a higher percentage of Baltimore-area operators were located in the city; in Cleveland, more were located in surrounding suburban counties. In Baltimore, significantly more African American op-erators than white operators were participants in the Project HOME pro-

Table 6

Characteristics of Board-and-Care Home Operators,
Baltimore and Cleveland

Characteristic	Cleveland (N = 139)	Baltimore (N = 103)
Mean age (yr)	50.9[a,b,c]	56.0[c]
(Range)	(23–74)	(32–77)
African American[d] (%)	29.5[b]	69.3[e]
Female (%)	91.4	98.1
Education		
Mean years school		10.95[c]
(Range)		(0–18)
High school + (%)	63.3[a]	
Marital status		
Married (%)	50.4[a,b]	43.1[a]
Widowed (%)	22.3	24.5
Divorced/separated (%)	23.0	27.5
Never married (%)	4.3	4.9
Self-rated health		
Fair (%)		21.4
Good (%)		53.4
Excellent (%)		25.2
Mean years providing care	7.2[c]	8.4[c]
(Range)	(0–30)	(0–39)
Other current employment (%)	15.1	25.5[c]

[a]Differences by race within sample statistically significant ($p < .05$).

[b]Differences by home size (1–3 vs. 4–8 residents) statistically significant ($p < .05$).

[c]Difference by average fee (above or below median) statistically significant ($p < .05$).

[d]Operators in Cleveland included only African American and white individuals, but the Baltimore sample included two Asians, who are excluded in race comparisons. African Americans include those of Caribbean origin.

[e]Difference by participation in Project HOME statistically significant ($p < .05$).

gram (52.2 percent and 28.6 percent, respectively). The informal networks (e.g., learning about board-and-care from family and friends) recruiting into Project HOME may be especially strong in the African American community. It is noteworthy, however, that the percentage of African American operators in both urban areas was higher than the percentage of African Americans in the general metropolitan population (Bureau of the Census 1993), suggesting that more individuals from the minority community were attracted to or find themselves in this type of work.

Data from both cities conformed with prior studies in that the great majority (91.4 percent in Cleveland and 98.1 percent in Baltimore) of home operators were women (Dittmar et al. 1983; Harmon 1982; Mor, Sherwood, and Gutkin 1986; Sherman and Newman 1988).

Education level was also fairly comparable for the two groups, with the average years of school completed by Baltimore operators approaching eleven years and nearly two-thirds of Cleveland operators having high school diplomas or more. Asking the actual years of schooling in Baltimore revealed a considerable range of education, from no formal schooling to postgraduate study (eighteen years completed). In Baltimore, the operators in higher-fee homes had more years of education; in Cleveland, there was a difference by race, with white operators having completed more schooling (see table 6). The educational attainment of operators had been shown to vary widely in a study of larger homes (Dittmar et al. 1983). In that study educational levels were somewhat higher than those found among our small board-and-care home operators and those in the most similar prior study by Sherman and Newman (1988).

Distributions by marital status were similar in Cleveland and Baltimore, except that slightly fewer of the Baltimore-area operators were married. This contrasts sharply with Sherman and Newman's samples, in which fewer than 6 percent of foster care providers were married (1988). In both of our operator samples, however, African Americans were more likely than whites to be widowed or divorced, and in Cleveland the operators of large homes were more likely to be married. This higher percentage of married operators in larger homes parallels the findings of other research (see Dittmar et al. 1983; Harmon 1982). Perhaps the presence of a spouse, through the assistance he provides, enables the care of a larger number of residents, an issue that is further addressed in chapter 6.

Using the OARS questions for self-rated health, most Baltimore-area operators rated their health as good or excellent, despite ages ranging into the seventies. There were no significant differences in self-reported health status by race, size of the home, or the level of fees being charged. Most of these operators (82.5 percent) confirmed that their health did not stand in the way ("at all") of doing the things they wanted to do and that their health was "about the same" (62.1 percent) or "better" (19.4 percent) than it had been five years earlier.

The average length of time providing care also varied widely among the operators, but the averages were similar for the samples in the two locations we studied. The average length of time in board-and-care work approached eight and one-half years for Baltimore operators and slightly over seven years for Cleveland-area operators. In both samples there was a difference by fee level, with the operators of lower-fee homes having provided care longer (4 years longer on average in Baltimore, 2.4 years longer in Cleveland). Whether this indicated the "staying power" of lower-fee homes (or of a few lower-fee providers) or the recent entry of higher-fee homes into the marketplace was not entirely clear. Data presented in table 6, showing that younger women tended to operate the higher-fee homes in both cities, support the latter argument.

Finally, as table 6 shows, more operators in Baltimore than in Cleveland held employment in addition to their board-and-care work. In Baltimore, employment differed neither by race nor by home size but was *more* common among operators of higher-fee homes. This unexpected result may simply reflect the fact that many residents in the Project HOME program, which subsidized fees into our high-fee range, also received day-care services. Presence of day programs then enabled operators to combine their caregiving with outside employment. This argument is partially supported by a difference in employment rates for operators in Project HOME (35.9 percent) and those who were not (18.1 percent), even though the difference did not achieve statistical significance.

Getting into the Business

A greater understanding of the operators and their characteristics comes from an examination of how and why they started offering board-and-care services. In both studies the operators were asked an open-ended question, "How did you start taking people into your home?" One or two responses were coded for each operator. In Baltimore, the five most commonly mentioned factors were suggestion from a friend or family member to undertake board-and-care (38.8 percent of operators), a desire to provide alternative housing (to nursing homes or mental institutions) (18.4 percent), an outgrowth of prior employment in health care (16.5 percent), the need for a job, and the receipt of information on board-and-care from the media or other sources (15.5 percent each). Additional answers from more than 10 percent of the Baltimore sample included having had experience caring for a family member or having done related work in the past.

In Cleveland, the most common response by far was having had prior experience with board-and-care work (53.2 percent). In this group, the recommendation of a friend or relative was the second most common reason for starting this work (20.2 percent), followed by economic necessity (18.7 percent), a desire to "try to help" (16.5 percent), and creation of a business (15.8 percent). No other answers were shared by more than 10 percent of Cleveland operators.

In both samples, recommendations of friends or family and prior experience, either in related health care or in board-and-care directly, were avenues to initiating board-and-care services. We also asked operators about prior employment and other experiences that may have served as pathways to provision of board-and-care. Among operators in Cleveland, 71.9 percent had previously worked in a hospital or nursing home, a figure that was remarkably consistent with the 69.9 percent of operators in Baltimore reporting prior work caring for the ill or infirm. Further questioning in Baltimore revealed a variety of prior jobs, including nurse aides, home health aides, and other health care occupations, mostly with low to moderate skill levels. In addition, more than half of the Baltimore operators (51.7 percent) revealed a family history of kin taking in other people or doing health care work in the community.

One criticism of operators of small homes has been their lack of training in areas such as bookkeeping, records management, and the interpretation and implementation of regulations (Dittmar and Smith 1983). In addition, the operators reported a variety of prior experiences and preparation before starting a board-and-care home. An open-ended question allowed Baltimore operators to provide up to three responses regarding education, training, or experience that had helped to prepare them for work in board-and-care. The most frequent response was having had a training course or program on caregiving (51.4 percent), although operators tended to mention it as a second or third response, rather than as their first answer. Although we might suspect this to be another result of the participation of a substantial number of Baltimore operators in Project HOME, which includes training as part of its program, the program participants were only slightly more likely than others to have given a response of training program to this question.

Other major responses included having cared for a relative (42.7 percent), prior work experience (35.9 percent), the completion of a certificate or degree in a related area (28.4 percent), and learning directly from physicians or other professionals (13.6 percent). Other, scattered responses included having taken college courses, having read or studied on their own, having raised children, having learned from other caregivers, or experience volunteering with elders. Clearly, the type of training and experience viewed by these small home operators as most relevant was related to direct care, not the business aspects of board-and-care mentioned by Dittmar and Smith (1983).

The avenues into board-and-care work, then, are not entirely governed by the formal mechanisms typical of many more professionalized health care fields. Not everyone has consistent education or formal training in preparation for the work, and a significant number of operators have come to this work through informal networks (recommendations of friends, family) and with variable training backgrounds. Again, the amalgam of formal and informal dimensions is clear in terms of the avenues into board-and-care careers.

Motivations and Rewards of Caregiving

Relatively few prior studies have examined the motivations for continuing in this type of work. A few studies of adult foster care and board-and-care homes found that "wanting to help someone else" was the most commonly stated reason for getting into this type of work, with the need for money mentioned about half as often (Braun, Horwitz, and Kaku 1988; Mor, Sherwood, and Gutkin 1986; Sherman and Newman 1988). Others (Feldman 1990; Holtz 1982) reinforced the desire to help as primary among the motivations for home health workers and nursing home aides, with pay ranking at the bottom. Kaye (1986) added affection received from clients as a factor in motivation, and others (Bartoldus, Gillery, and Sturges 1989; Gubrium 1975; Holtz 1982) suggested religious motivations.

In the first Baltimore interview, operators were asked, "What are the main benefits and rewards you gain from continuing to run this home?" Up to three answers were coded from each operator's open-ended responses. By far the most frequent answer was that operators liked to help people (73.8 percent). Beyond that response, other altruistic motivations also appeared. Operators mentioned liking the company of their residents (12.6 percent), rewards from helping people avoid nursing home placement (14.6 percent), being gratified when clients did well (18.4 percent), and enjoying their clients (20.4 percent). Not all responses were altruistic, however, since about one operator in four (25.2 percent) mentioned economic rewards or motivations for operating the home.

Additional attitude items, interspersed in the caregiver burden scale, attempted to evaluate the orientations of the operators toward their work. These items were notable by the strong agreement in the responses (using a five-point Likert-type response format, in which 5 indicates "strongly agree"). For three of these five questions, all responses were in the neutral to strongly agree range; for the two remaining items, only one operator responded in a negative manner. Because of this positive skew in the responses, only those "strongly agreeing" with each statement are noted. These items included "I really enjoy spending time with the clients" (68 percent strongly agree); "The happiness of clients over some little things I do gives me pleasure" (90.3 percent strongly agree); "Knowing you are doing your best gets you through the rough times" (79.6 percent strongly agree); "I enjoy my work, because it is helping these people" (85.4 percent strongly agree); and "I am pleased to help some people stay out of nursing homes" (86.4 percent strongly agree). We concluded that the operators strongly identified with the interpersonal aspects of their work and that these aspects may provide gratifications that encourage them to continue in board-and-care work.

The altruistic motivations of helping others reappeared throughout our discussions with the board-and-care home operators. One Baltimore operator summed it up for many when she said, "I've always given someone a home." She just considered it a natural thing to do. "Everybody needs a home—needs to belong to a family setting. People should care for others that need it."

Burden of Caregiving in Small Board-and-Care Homes

Considerable research attention has focused on caregiver burden, primarily among family members assisting frail kin in the community (Ory et al. 1985; Pearson, Sumer, and Nellett 1988). This family-based research has now moved beyond simple notions of burden by focusing on its multidimensionality, identifying several themes or domains of burden in these caregiving relationships (George and Gwyther 1986; Novak and Guest 1989).

The operators of small board-and-care homes demonstrate important similarities to and differences from both family caregivers and paraprofessionals such as nursing home aides. While the physical demands of caring may be higher in board-and-care homes for operators who must assist a larger number of individuals with multiple impairments than they are for family caregivers, the operators' background, experience, and training, as well as some emotional distance may ease the strains of caregiving. In contrast to other paid caregivers, however, the small board-and-care home operators share a twenty-four-hour responsibility for those in their care.

Surprisingly little research attention has been directed to the problem of burden among paraprofessionals providing intense direct care to multiple frail elders on a daily basis (Chappell and Novak 1992). Those studies that do exist give mixed views, with some showing limited burden (Bartoldus, Gillery, and Sturges 1989; Dillard and Feather 1989) and others suggesting much higher levels (Chandler, Rachal, and Kazelskis 1986; Chappell and Novak 1992). Given the reliance on operators as primary caregivers to multiple dependent adults, one major concern of the Baltimore study was the degree to which, and the conditions under which, operators of small homes experienced burden.

When asked whether they had ever considered ceasing the operation of board-and-care, about one in five Baltimore operators said yes. Primary among the reasons were issues related to burnout (e.g., feeling worn out, no relief from the stress of caregiving, clients being too much work). Thus, the issue of burnout appears to be of importance in the eyes of the operators themselves as a reason that operators quit.

How We Evaluated Burden

A scale of twenty-three items to measure burden was developed from questions in prior studies, augmented by others created specifically for this population. The resulting scale was administered as part of each operator interview in Baltimore. Responses were Likert-style, varying from 5 ("strongly agree") to 1 ("strongly disagree"). The items described earlier on rewards of caregiving were interspersed with the burden items to avoid response-set bias. Four dimensions of burden were hypothesized to be relevant to these operators: physical, psychological, financial, and time/privacy (Novak and Guest 1989). The underlying concept of concern was the perceived or subjective level of burden, assumed to affect operators negatively in their work (Montgomery, Stull, and Borgatta 1985; Morycz 1980; Poulshock and Deimling 1984).

Examples of items in the psychological dimension (five items) include, "Caring for people in my home has made me nervous or anxious" and "The work I do is mentally draining or exhausting." Physical health items (five) included "Running a board-and-care home sometimes takes more physical effort than I can give" and "I am generally very tired as a result of caring for the clients." The time and privacy dimension, containing eight items, included such statements as "It's hard to plan things ahead when the clients needs are so unpredictable," "My work here usually takes away too much time from other things I would like to do," and "Caring for the people living here doesn't give me as much privacy as I would like." Finally, the financial dimension (five items) contained items such as "I don't earn enough money for the amount of work that I do" and "I worry a lot about the costs of running this home."

An evaluation of the measurement properties of the twenty-three-item additive scale showed adequate reliability (α ranged from .822 to .897 across various interviews). Subscales reflecting the dimensions also demonstrated adequate reliability ($\alpha = .552$ to .854).

Trends in Burden among Operators

Perhaps the most surprising result was that the operators of small board-and-care homes reported fairly low levels of burden, using questions similar to those employed for family caregivers. Table 7 outlines the basic scores for the total scale and for each dimension over time. First, examining the total burden scores in a scale ranging from 23 to 115 points, additive scores

Table 7

Caregiving Burden among Baltimore Home Operators:
Scores for Dimensions and Changes over Time

	Mean	S.D.	Range	α	Correlations* with		
					Time 2	Time 3	Time 4
Time 1							
Burden (N = 100)[a]	51.1	15.5	23–115	.888	.683	.710	.693
Emotional	8.9	3.6	5–25	.689	.487	.567	.576
Physical	8.2	3.7	5–25	.700	.495	.603	.546
Financial	14.1	5.1	5–25	.693	.607	.646	.576
Time/privacy	19.6	6.7	8–40	.816	.671	.672	.656
Time 2							
Burden (N = 87)	52.6	12.5	23–115	.822		.744	.669
Emotional	9.5	3.2	5–25	.552		.613	.446
Physical	8.6	3.4	5–25	.662		.646	.546
Financial	14.2	4.6	5–25	.664		.681	.654
Time/privacy	20.3	6.0	8–40	.764		.738	.731
Time 3							
Burden (N = 87)	53.1	14.6	23–115	.878			.778
Emotional	9.2	3.1	5–25	.565			.655
Physical	9.0	3.8	5–25	.731			.734
Financial	14.2	4.7	5–25	.668			.740
Time/privacy	20.4	6.9	8–40	.842			
Time 4							
Burden (N = 89)	54.9	15.2	23–115	.897			
Emotional	9.6	3.5	5–25	.697			
Physical	9.6	3.7	5–25	.757			
Financial	14.6	5.0	5–25	.764			
Time/privacy	21.0	6.9	8–40	.854			

[a]N indicates the minimum number of respondents completing any of the subscales in that set of interviews.

*Correlations are statistically significant ($p < .01$).

were in the low to mid 50s, indicating that burden is not a major problem in the operator population. Examination of the individual items showed that few of them even approached majority agreement (data not shown), but operators and individual items varied widely. The reliability for the total scale was high, and mean scores were fairly consistent across all four interviews. Not only did the mean scores remain consistent, but also individual operators' scores were predictive of their subsequent scores, as shown by the consistently strong and significant correlations.

The topical subscales showed that operators felt the most burdened in the financial area. Mean scores for that subscale, relative to its range, were substantially higher in all four interviews than those for the other three areas evaluated. Again, the reliabilities were high and subscale scores were predictive of later measurements on those same items. Perhaps surprisingly, given the nature of the work, operators did not report significant burden in physical, emotional, and time/privacy areas. Additional analyses showed that burden scores for operators had significant, but only modest (.31 or less), correlations with the levels of resident impairment. Burden was also correlated with operator depression ($r = .40$ with the CES-D index), and the number of residents ($r = .268$) and negatively correlated with operator age ($r = -.242$) and years of operation ($r = -.167$).

An open-ended question in the Baltimore study, placed just before the burden scale, asked operators "What is the one thing about caring for your clients that causes you the most physical problem or mental stress?" Most of the operators gave some response, with twenty-six distinct answers coded. The most common response, given by nearly one-quarter (24.7 percent), related to stresses arising from client behavior problems. Following that, multiple responses appeared for client illnesses (8.2 percent), heavy reliance of residents on the operator, resident resistance to hygiene, and incontinence (5.9 percent each). Other responses, including a lack of improvement in clients, medication problems, a lack of privacy, conflict among clients, financial limitations, and the operator's inability to help enough, were mentioned by three or fewer operators.

Examples of the feelings of burden and stress were provided in comments made to our interviewers. One operator admitted that she felt a "personal strain" since she had started taking people into her home, seeing herself as a "security blanket" to the clients. "I really feel a heavy weight of responsibility in taking care of these people. They look up to me. They rely on me. They see me as a very strong person who is their protector. Sometimes I don't think I can do everything that they expect from me. The clients and my family have built up an image of me that I just don't think I can always live up to."

Why Burden Is/Isn't a Problem

Finding the generally low level of burden overall and only modest associations with variables we might expect to influence it raises important questions. In light of others' findings of substantial burden among family members providing care for frail elders at home, why did these paraprofessional operators not demonstrate comparable levels of strain or burden?

One obvious possibility is the fundamental difference in the nature of the relationship to the person receiving care. The absence of long-term emotional bonds and shared history enables operators to conceptualize the caregiving they perform in a fashion that shields them from some of the stresses of family caregivers. Since operators conceptualize this as their work, rather than as something to be added to an existing schedule of work and family responsibilities (as it is among kin providing care), the underlying expectations are different. Although, as we shall see, most of them consider their residents to be "just like family," there remains a difference of possibly critical importance in the links between caregiver and care recipient. They may, in fact, practice "detached attachment," enabling them to maintain some essential emotional distance from those they assist (Nelson 1990).

A second potential difference is the chosen nature of the caregiving situation. Operators of small board-and-care homes choose to perform this type of work, although some might argue about the freedom of their "choice" (Enarson 1990). Family members, in contrast, face an obligation or duty to provide care that is inherent in their roles as spouse or child (Brody et al. 1983; Brody, Kleban, and Johnson 1987). This spousal or filial duty requires that individuals fulfill the caregiving responsibilities regardless of their abilities or preference. Operators of homes, on the other hand, have chosen this type of work. Those who find the responsibilities too daunting or who are uncomfortable with the demands on their time and privacy have the option of ceasing board-and-care work. For most operators, such a decision would necessitate taking other employment, but most of them have worked in other settings before (or concurrently with) their board-and-care work. A return to a more traditional working environment might limit the burden associated with twenty-four-hour care in the home. Thus, board-and-care home providers are a self-selected group, in contrast to kin who act as caregivers.

A third potential explanation has to do with the operators' recognition of their own limitations in caring for residents. For both studies, most homes were legally unlicensed, so no agency placed constraints on the level or type of impairments among the residents taken into them (Kane, Wilson, and Clemmer 1993). Thus, operators were left to determine whether a particular applicant was acceptable and, on the other end, when someone became too ill or difficult for them to keep (see also chap. 5). In both studies, operators were asked if there were particular types of clients they would not accept. Research with state agency personnel (Hawes et al. 1993) suggested that persons with mental and cognitive illnesses (especially those who were disruptive), those with substance abuse problems, and those receiving SSI were difficult to place in board-and-care homes.

Anecdotal information given to our interviewers during in-depth discussions suggested that these limitations often arose for operators after a difficult experience with a particular type of resident. In the Cleveland survey, operators were given a list of types of clients and asked whether they would be willing to accept someone of that type. In Baltimore, rather than structuring the responses, operators were asked in an open-ended format, "For whatever reasons, what kinds of clients are you currently not willing to accept?" Many of their responses mirrored those given by the Cleveland operators, but others augmented the original list. Not surprisingly, since the responses were volunteered in answer to an open-ended question, all percentages are lower for the Baltimore sample, with the exception of those unacceptable types of resident that were not listed in the Cleveland question. The results are summarized in figures 14 through 16.

Categories (behavioral, physical, and cognitive/mental) were used to organize the responses, although the items did not appear under these headings in the Cleveland interview instrument. Although there are more physical problems listed, the percentages of operators mentioning particular types of residents as unacceptable are higher in the behavioral and cognitive/mental areas. First, in the behavioral category a strong majority (87.7 percent) of Cleveland operators were unwilling to accept problem drinkers (as were 22.3 percent of Baltimore operators), with fewer than half as many (38.8 percent) unwilling to accept occasional drinkers. Smaller but important percentages of operators reported an unwillingness to accept young adults (43.2 percent) and smokers (28.8 percent). The Baltimore

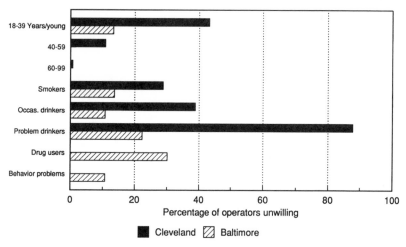

Fig. 14. Percentage of Operators Unwilling to Accept Particular Types of Residents: Behavioral Problems

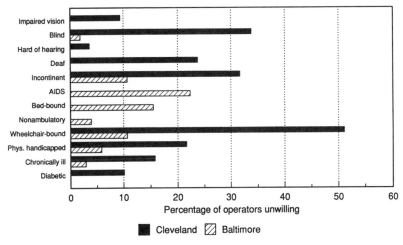

Fig. 15. Percentage of Operators Unwilling to Accept Particular Types of Residents: Physical Problems

operators added drug users (30.1 percent) and residents with serious behavioral problems (10.7 percent) to the list of those unacceptable because of behavior problems.

Turning to physical problems, those most likely to be unacceptable to Cleveland operators were wheelchair-bound (51.1 percent), blind (33.8

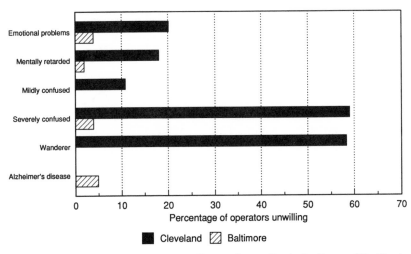

Fig. 16. Percentage of Operators Unwilling to Accept Particular Types of Residents: Cognitive and Mental Problems

percent), incontinent (31.7 percent), deaf (23.7 percent), or physically handicapped (21.6 percent) residents. Concerns of the Baltimore operators were highest for a category not listed in Cleveland (probably because of timing), the resident with AIDS. Nearly one-quarter of Baltimore operators (22.3 percent) mentioned being unwilling to accept AIDS patients as residents. Also of note were those who were bed-bound (15.5 percent), incontinent (10.7 percent), or wheelchair-bound (10.7 percent). One operator, after reporting her unwillingness to accept an AIDS client, explained, "I know these people would die, and I don't think I could deal with them dying."

Cognitive/mental problems were also reasons for nonacceptance, with nearly six in ten of the Cleveland operators unwilling to accept severely confused or wandering residents. Much greater acceptance was found for those with emotional problems, retardation, or mild confusion. Operators in the Baltimore sample mirrored many of these concerns, adding Alzheimer's disease, which may subsume many of the "wanderers" mentioned by Cleveland operators.

In addition to those conditions listed in figures 14 through 16, a few (one to three) Baltimore operators also mentioned being unwilling to accept those with a colostomy or who were oxygen dependent, had serious skin problems, or used canes. Operators in both cities also made distinctions based on residents' sex and race, with more not accepting men than women (17.3 percent in Cleveland, compared with Baltimore's 7.9 percent), and fewer white operators accepting those of a different race, as will be quite apparent in chapter 5. In all, operators seemed very willing to identify problems with residents that made them unacceptable, perhaps recognizing their own limitations in caring for persons with particular needs.

Unmet Needs Reported by Operators

Despite the modest level of reported burden, operators were not without problems. Both studies inquired about problems faced by the operators. First, an open-ended question to Cleveland operators asked, "What problems do you encounter in running this facility?" A comparable question in Baltimore asked, "What problems have you had in the past year in running this home and caring for clients?" The results of the top five responses for each operator sample (and the corresponding results for the same problem in the other urban area's sample) are listed on figure 17. It is noteworthy that while many operators did report one or more problem, the types of problems reported were widely scattered, with most categories in each sample mentioned by fewer than one in ten operators. Also, most of the

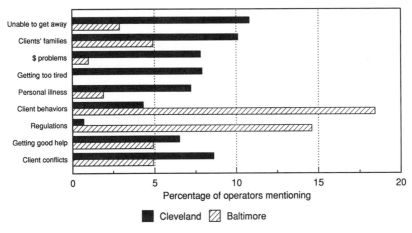

Fig. 17. Leading Problems Identified by Board-and-Care Home Operators
Note: Slightly different questions were used for the two samples.

problems mentioned in the top five in each area were mentioned by at least some operators in the other sample, indicating similar themes emerging in terms of the difficulties faced by operators in daily operation. Many of the problems discovered in these samples also reflect those described elsewhere as problematic to board-and-care providers (Reisacher 1989).

The most frequently mentioned issue among Baltimore operators was behavior problems of clients; almost one in five (18.4 percent) mentioned such difficulties. The fact that few in the Cleveland operator sample mentioned this type of problem may reinforce the differences brought about by the presence of the Project HOME program in Maryland, which places many deinstitutionalized mental patients. In a parallel vein, Baltimore operators were much more likely to mention problems with regulation or conflict with regulations (14.6 percent) than were the Cleveland operators (0.7 percent). Further detail regarding the problems that Baltimore operators experienced with regulation in their political environments is included below.

Top problems among the Cleveland operators included the difficulty in getting away from client-care responsibilities (10.8 percent), problems with client families (10.1 percent), and conflicts with the clients themselves (8.6 percent). Again, smaller percentages of Baltimore-area operators mentioned these same problems with the family members of residents. Additional problems that operators mentioned included financial problems, getting too tired, personal illness, and getting or retaining good helpers to work in the board-and-care home or to provide respite.

Specific Problems of Home Operation

We followed up in greater detail on several areas that were problematic to operators. These areas include training, unmet needs for assistance and support, problems in locating residents and filling vacancies, respite, and regulations and regulators.

Training

We asked Baltimore operators whether they thought their training and experience was "enough to prepare you for the work you do every day in caring for clients?" and what additional training "might help you now in caring for your clients or running your board-and-care home?" A strong majority of Baltimore-area operators (92.7 percent) said that their background was sufficient, in their view, to prepare them for board-and-care work.

Responses to the open-ended question on additional training desired now included training regarding medications (13.6 percent), the management of mental health problems (11.7 percent), courses on caregiving (8.7 percent), administrative or business aspects of operating the home (7.8 percent), and information on physical or mental health conditions of clients (7.8 percent). Inadequate training on medications has been a specific criticism of the staff in small board-and-care homes (GAO 1992). Less frequently mentioned responses included dealing with burnout or burden, learning about activities and recreation, and safety or licensure regulations. The largest response (37.9 percent) was that no additional training would be of help currently.

Unmet Needs for Help

In the first Baltimore interview operators were asked "What other types of help do you need that you are not getting in caring for clients or running the home?" Almost half of the operators (47.6 percent) had no response, and most of the remainder (31.1 percent) gave one unmet need. A few operators (4.9 percent) reported three types of additional unmet needs. Most-often mentioned was the need for respite (13.6 percent) or reliable backup caregivers (4.9 percent), followed by needing more money for residents (10.7 percent). Other needs mentioned by a few caregivers included resources for activities or recreation, help in locating clients, money to expand their board-and-care operation, assistance with mental health care of clients, and aid in providing religious services.

Locating/Replacing Residents

A problem mentioned by a significant number of operators was that of locating appropriate clients for their homes when a vacancy occurred. This problem is apparently common in small homes (McCoin 1983). Prior research suggests that residents come to board-and-care through a variety of formal and informal referral mechanisms (see chap. 5) (Dittmar et al. 1983). The "mirror image" problem, potential residents and their families having difficulty locating homes, also appears in the literature (Harmon 1982). More than one-quarter of Baltimore-area operators (27.0 percent) reported having had a period of time without any residents since they started providing board-and-care services. For most operators this clientless period was relatively brief, with 25.9 percent recalling spans of three or fewer months without clients, and two-thirds (66.7 percent) of these spans lasted a year or less. One-third of operators attributed such gaps to the inability to locate residents, with more than one in four (25.9 percent) blaming it on the death of resident(s), and slightly fewer (22.2 percent) claiming unacceptable residents as the core of the problem.

Most operators in Baltimore (87.3 percent) also claimed that they would seek to fill a vacancy if one occurred at the time of the interview, with their most important reasons for doing so being the availability of space (30.1 percent), people needing a home (21.4 percent), wanting to help (21.4 percent), and improved atmosphere and morale in the home with more clients in residence (10.7 percent). Strategies for filling vacancies also varied among operators. When operators were asked how they went about filling vacancies, their open-ended responses most often involved contacting referral agencies (47.6 percent), hospitals (18.4 percent), and social workers (16.5 percent). Fewer operators relied on such strategies as newspaper advertisement, personal contacts, and advising local churches or physicians.

Respite

Given the problematic nature of respite for many operators in Cleveland, the Baltimore study included a number of detailed questions to examine this area. Surprisingly, the Baltimore operators were somewhat less likely to see respite as a serious problem. Of this group, only 6.7 percent said respite was always or usually a problem for them, 16.9 percent said it was sometimes a problem, and 76.4 percent said it was seldom or never a problem. Both African American operators and those who were affiliated with Project HOME were significantly less likely to report respite as a serious problem, but there were no significant differences by home size or fees paid by residents. Again, part of the difference in the two studies may arise from the presence of Project HOME in Baltimore. Operators who participated in that program were significantly less likely to report respite as a problem (76.9 percent answered that respite was "never a problem," compared with 45.8 percent of nonparticipants). The program's requirement for backup caregivers apparently prompted participants to address this issue before it became a problem for them.

When we asked these same operators about the availability of respite caregivers for short time periods (one to two hours), full days, or weekends or longer periods, we were somewhat surprised by the responses. Only two operators claimed to have no respite providers they could rely on for short time periods, a figure that grew to seven and nine operators for the full day and weekend or longer alternatives, respectively. Most operators listed one or more respite caregivers, and the numbers of persons they could call on ranged up to twelve. The bulk of the operators, however, reported numbers toward the low end of the distribution. For example, 59.3 percent claimed one to three persons available to them for short-term respite, with a similar figure (58.3 percent) for full-day respite, and more (63.1 percent) reporting one to three backup caregivers for weekends or longer periods of time. Perhaps not surprisingly, relatives of the operator were most commonly called upon to provide respite care, followed by friends.

Most operators in Baltimore (62.9 percent) reported using respite for both leisure activities and necessary trips outside the board-and-care home, but some (22.5 percent) said they restricted respite to only necessary trips. Three-quarters (77.5 percent) said that they paid their respite caregivers for their services, but most (61.7 percent) said the cost did not keep them from going out when they wished or needed to do so. Costs for respite care varied widely, depending on the time period for which payment was made. One operator reported paying a maximum of $325 per month for respite, while weekly fees ranged from $55 to $240. Daily and hourly fees varied as well, with daily rates ranging from $5 to $50 and hourly rates from $3 to $10. Depending on the frequency of use, respite is potentially an expensive item for many operators.

When the Baltimore operators were asked in an open-ended format (with up to two responses coded) what else they did (in addition to or in lieu of payment) to compensate backup caregivers, they gave a variety of responses. Of those responding ($N = 79$), half said that they reciprocated by doing things for the respite caregiver (50.6 percent); giving gifts (25.3 percent); or giving them things, including goods, meals, or housing (20.3 percent); while 24.0 percent said they did nothing. These bartering exchanges for respite services are quite understandable since many of those giving such care are relatives, perhaps including those sharing the household.

Finding someone to care for clients so she could get away was a frequent problem for one atypical Baltimore operator. Although she could do many necessary tasks while her residents were at day-care, in emergencies she relied on her sister, who also had young children, to cover her clients.

Recently she tried to find someone so that she and her family could take a vacation. Since one client had become incontinent, she learned that it would cost $125 per day to provide care, contrasted with the $50 per day she had paid before. "We shouldn't have to rely on newspaper ads [to find respite caregivers]—then you have to worry about the clients *and* your home."

Regulation and Regulators

Limited attention has been paid to the role of regulators and regulations in the smaller board-and-care home (Dobkin 1989). A small study of adult foster care (Braun, Horwitz, and Kaku 1988) found that most operators viewed the level of staff supervision in their program as "just right." Since details regarding the interview situation in that study were lacking, it is unclear whether social desirability influenced the responses. Others (Feder et al. 1989) have suggested that operators actively avoid external oversight, sometimes preferring to think that they know what is best for their "families."

In the fourth Baltimore interview, questions were included to tap the operators' experience of and attitude toward regulation and regulators. The first item asked operators about regulators or agencies that had visited, called, or sent them something during the past year because of the board-and-care home. Of the ninety operators responding to this interview, seventy-seven reported at least one such contact, and fifty-one reported three or more. Among the agencies or groups most commonly in contact with the operators were the health department (63.3 percent), the fire department (64.4 percent), and Project HOME (44.4 percent). Other groups visiting a small percentage of operators included the local social services agency, Adult Protective Services, the Office on Aging, the Department of Health and Mental Hygiene, the Veteran's Administration, and the police. The great majority of the groups visited or were in contact only once during the year, but visits ranged up to several times a month in some instances. The purpose of most visits was to monitor the home (e.g., annual inspections) or for routine oversight of its residents, with fewer visits involving client problems or coordinating services for the home's residents.

Since most homes in the Baltimore sample are considered "unregulated" by virtue of not being involved in a state licensure program, the volume and variety of their contact with regulatory agencies is impressive. Among homes not participating in Project HOME, more than one in four (26.5 percent) reported no contact with a regulator in the prior year, and their median number of regulator contacts was one or two. Project HOME operators, on the other hand, all reported contact with at least one and an average of three regulatory agencies or persons during that same time period. The frequency of visits by agencies, however, was quite similar for the two groups.

In light of the contact with regulatory and oversight groups, we asked operators whether "people from governmental agencies [should] have anything to say about how you operate your home?" Nearly three of four Baltimore operators (72.2 percent) responded positively. Almost the same percentage (74.1 percent) characterized people from government agencies as having been "mostly helpful" to them in the past year, in contrast to the more negative contentions of Feder and associates (1989).

But the Baltimore operator sample was not entirely uncritical. When we asked whether there were ways in which these regulators and their agencies could be more helpful, 41.7 percent responded in the affirmative. A follow-up question (open-ended) asked how they might do better. Responses ranged from "leave me alone" to aiding in the resolution of conflicts with clients, providing more money for care, improving client services, and improving communication with agencies. None of the categories received more than a few responses, but several focused on the theme of money (more money for the care provided, money for client recreation, spending money for clients, money for client damage to the home or its contents).

One Baltimore operator had recently received a letter from a regulatory agency informing her of unannounced visits. "I understand that it is their right, but this is *my home!* I don't let anyone in my house unannounced—family, friend, *no one* has the right to invade my privacy." She was apparently so distressed by this policy that she was considering ending her years as a care provider. Another operator described her years of fighting with legislators for laws to protect operators and recognize the good care given in small homes. Having given up on the passage of such provisions, she plans to close her home as soon as her debt, undertaken to meet state specifications, is paid off in three years.

In referring to "the authorities," another operator stated that they were putting pressure on her to "get licensed." She said, "They made me feel like a criminal." She noted that the fire department told her she needed a sprinkler system, but "the program, the State" said that this was not required. One operator, who had spent time advocating for board-and-care services, felt that her efforts were not appreciated and that she was not given any respect by legislators or regulators. In particular, she was frustrated by the restrictions placed on her regarding the administration of medications, tending to decubitus ulcers, and other health needs of the residents.

Ways to Assist Board-and-Care Home Operators

In an earlier report, Harmon (1982) listed a variety of actions that might enhance the operation of small board-and-care homes, enabling operators to maintain their service while improving the quality of care and oversight. Included in Harmon's list were encouraging provider associations, imposing financial penalties for noncompliance with regulations (rather than closing down beds), providing technical assistance to operators to meet regulatory and service guidelines, providing grants and loans to operators to finance modifications to meet standards, and working with the private sector to reduce the costs of board-and-care services in some areas. She also suggested increasing linkages to services for residents in board-and-care homes and programs to guarantee the recruitment and training of new operators over time.

Several similar items were included in the third interview with Baltimore operators. The responses from operators are summarized in figure 18. Operator endorsement of the listed alternatives as important to assist them in their work ranged from three-quarters down to about one-quarter of those responding.

Among the supports viewed as helpful by the largest percentages, a referral system to locate clients (66.7 percent), better financial support to care for clients (64.4 percent), and respite care (63.3 percent) were the most popular. Less commonly endorsed, but still favored by over half of operators, were training courses on caring for people (56.7 percent), low-cost home-improvement loans, better health care services for clients, and more and better day-care services (supported by 51.1 percent each). Least impor-

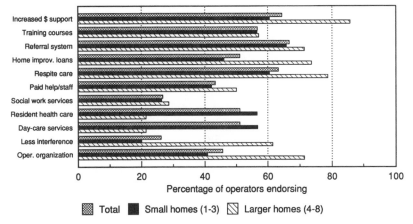

Fig. 18. Approval of Various Supports to Their Work by Baltimore Home Operators

tant in the view of the Baltimore operators were reducing interference from the authorities (26.1 percent) and providing more social work services for clients (26.7 percent).

There were only limited differences on these items by the characteristics of the home and its operator. No significant differences appeared by fee level, and only one was apparent by race. African American operators were more likely to support improved day-care services for their clients (58.3 percent approved) as an important goal. Five of the items had significant differences by home size, as shown in figure 18. Operators in larger homes were more likely to support low-cost home improvement, less interference from authorities, and developing an operator organization, but were significantly less supportive of improving health care and day care services for residents.

Caregiver Success: The Operator's Perspective

To better understand how the operators themselves conceive of the important aspects of their roles and the skills to support their performance of that role, Baltimore operators responded to the open-ended question, "Based on your own experience and that of others you have known, what traits, skills, and abilities does an operator need to enjoy operating a good quality board-and-care home for a long time?" This question encouraged the operators to define the traits that they saw as central to successful performance of the provider role. The findings, from up to four open-ended responses from each operator, are summarized in the first column of table 8.

The most commonly mentioned trait was patience or understanding (48.9 percent), followed closely by having a caring attitude (tender loving care, or "TLC") (47.7 percent). Beyond these two responses, however, there is a major drop to the next set of items, including liking the work (22.2 percent), being compassionate (18.9 percent), and having good health, skill in caring for elders, and liking people (14.4 percent each). Being organized and efficient (13.3 percent) and having health care skills (12.2 percent) round out the characteristics mentioned spontaneously by at least one in ten of the responding operators.

There were some variations in the types of operators mentioning the various traits. White operators were more likely to mention having high energy, skill in working with elders, family support, compassion, and a good mind or education than were their African American counterparts. African American operators, for their part, more often mentioned a caring attitude or TLC as important to operator success. Operators caring for four to eight residents more often mentioned self-knowledge as important, and

Table 8

Baltimore Operators' Views of the Traits of Successful Operators, Interviewer Evaluations, and Operator Self-Evaluations

Trait	Operators Mentioning (%)	Ratings (% Excellent)		Correlation
		Interviewers	Operator/Self	
Patience/under-standing	48.9	51.1	57.8	.387*
Caring attitude/TLC	47.7[a]	58.3	74.4	.305*
Likes the work	22.2	70.5	80.0	.318*
Compassionate	18.9[a]	65.8	72.2	.257*
Good health/emotional strength	14.4	43.3[b]	38.2	.382*
Skilled with elders	14.4[a]	53.0	71.1	.146
Likes people	14.4	65.6[c]	90.0	−.021
Organized/efficient	13.3	51.7	45.6	.219*
Health care skills	12.2[b]	31.4	51.1	.139
Motivation	7.7	68.9	48.9	.388*
Hard work/dependability	5.5	81.1	71.6	.067
Sense of humor	5.5	42.2	62.9	.047
Knows how to set limits	4.4	55.6	48.9	.108
Knows herself	4.4[c]	64.4	71.9[a]	.214*
Good mind and education	3.3[a]	48.9[b]	53.3	.114
Lots of energy	2.2[a]	42.2	41.1[b]	.549*
Family support/participation	2.2[a]	47.1[b]	60.0	.434*
Adaptable/flexible to demands	2.2	41.2	46.7	.272*

[a]Difference by race statistically significant ($p < .05$).
[b]Difference by fee level statistically significant ($p < .05$).
[c]Differences by home size statistically significant ($p < .05$).
*Correlation significant ($p < .05$).

operators of higher-fee homes focused more on health care skills as key to success.

Since this profile of operator strengths emerged from those providing the care themselves, the items were subsequently used as a template for two sets of questions on caregiver performance in the fourth interview. Although these evaluations are admittedly subjective, the extremely sparse data available on quality of care prompted this examination (Reschovsky and Ruchlin 1993). In addition, subjective evaluations can sometimes be illuminating in and of themselves. First, we asked interviewers to rate the operators on these same characteristics, (with 4 representing "excellent," 1, "poor"). Next, we asked the operators to rate themselves on each of these eighteen somewhat overlapping aspects of caregiver quality or success, using the same rating scale. The results of those evaluations are reported in the second (interviewer ratings) and third (operator self-ratings) columns of table 8.

Turning first to interviewer ratings, it was clear that the views of interviewers with regard to the quality of work of the operators was high overall. The percentages in the table reflected only those marked "excellent," and on over half of these items a majority of operators were so rated. The highest percentage receiving excellent ratings was for hard work/dependability (81.1 percent), and the lowest percentage rated excellent occurred for health care skills, where nearly one-third (31.4 percent) of operators were still rated excellent.

There were some variations in how the interviewers rated operators, although relatively few statistically significant differences appeared. African American operators were more likely to be rated by their interviewers as "excellent" on the dimension of liking people. Operators in larger homes were more often rated as having excellent family support. Those operators in higher-fee homes were also rated better on the health/strength dimension and on having a good mind and education.

Operator self-ratings follow in the third column of table 8. It was clear from the responses we received that the operators were confident of their skills and resources to perform board-and-care work. Their self-ratings were higher, in most cases, than the interviewer ratings. The great majority of them rated themselves excellent with regard to liking people (90.0 percent), liking their work (80.0 percent), having a caring attitude (74.4 percent), knowing themselves (71.9 percent), hard work/dependability (71.6 percent), and being skilled with elders (71.1 percent). There were few variations among operators in our comparison groups (i.e., size of home, operator race, and level of fees) on these self-ratings, with the only exceptions being that African American operators more often rated themselves excellent in having lots of energy and knowing themselves.

Finally, table 8 shows the correlations between the interviewer's rating and the operator's self-rating on the same item. Many of the correlations were significant, and several approached moderate levels (with correlation sizes statistically constrained by the four-point rating scales on which each item was evaluated). Yet on several of the items the interviewers and the operators did not agree. This may have important implications for regulatory oversight in the home, if "outsiders" do not view the circumstances inside the home in the same way as the operator. Nonetheless, the overall evaluations of the skills and success of Baltimore-area home operators were quite positive. Both they and the interviewers considered them to be doing an excellent job in most respects.

Characteristics of the Job and Worker Satisfaction: Some Hypotheses

Motivating and maintaining a supply of board-and-care home operators, should society determine this care option worthy of support, raises issues of job satisfaction. Recruiting and motivating workers to provide direct service in a high-quality fashion necessitates creating or enhancing aspects of the job that provide satisfaction to workers. Existing theory on job satisfaction, including some relatively new ideas in this area, provide some potential explanations for the apparently strong motivations of board-and-care providers in the face of low fees, troublesome residents, and high levels of role ambiguity deriving from social marginality. Two such concepts are described here: Friedson's notion of "labors of love" and new views on alienation in the workplace.

Labors of Love: A Different View of Work

Classic writing about job satisfaction describes these satisfactions as either intrinsic or extrinsic. Extrinsic factors are most generally the objective rewards, such as pay and benefits, attached to particular jobs. Intrinsic rewards are the personal gratifications derived from doing a good job, seeing positive results from the work efforts, and similar intangible or subjective gratifications. This literature, as Friedson (1990) points out, tends to view work negatively, as an unpleasant necessity to be minimized by workers who can afford to do so.

Friedson suggests, in contrast to this negative view, that it is possible for work to be both creative and satisfying. He describes a special kind of work, which he dubs "labors of love," in which the task is freely chosen, part of the worker's nature, high in self-fulfillment, and motivated by factors other than purely economic ones (1990). Friedson criticizes our association of the definition of work with economic exchange, which fails to allow for altruism or love of the task undertaken. He proposes a broader definition of work, inclusive of all activity with use-value, not just exchange-value. Under this definition, labors of love are voluntarily chosen work that does not necessarily gain a living for its participant (Friedson 1990).

The operation of small board-and-care homes demonstrates some of the aspects of Friedson's concept of "labors of love," in that operators sometimes perform the work without significant economic gain. It is voluntarily chosen, with those unhappy with the work able to cease operation and turn to other employment. The operators repeatedly emphasized to our interviewers, in both formal responses and side comments, their commitment to the task of providing care. Altruistic motivations drove many to work at board-and-care, even though they had health limitations or were advancing in age. Many operators clearly identified who they were by the work they did in providing board-and-care services. They received a high level of gratification from their work and reported little burden, despite the unrelenting nature of the tasks at hand.

Alienation and the "McDonaldization" of Work

Another theme in the literature on work satisfaction is the Marxian issue of alienation, whereby individuals who are workers are separated from the satisfaction of seeing a complete task or product at the end of their work effort (Erikson 1990). The manufacturing focus of Marx's theory aside, more-contemporary theorists propose that the alienation of the workplace today comes about from the subdivision of work into narrower and narrower subspecialties or tasks and from limits on worker autonomy (Erikson 1990).

Efforts to increase the efficiency of work often focus on increasing rationalization, dividing work into smaller, specialized tasks that can be measured, timed, and efficiently recorded and evaluated to establish levels of performance (Ritzer 1993). Ritzer (1993), who sees this process, which he dubbed "McDonaldizing," occurring in most of corporate America, emphasizes that it permits employers to at least perceive that they are enhancing the efficiency, calculability, predictability, and control over their workers and the products or services they produce.

An example of this process in the service sector is provided by Diamond (1990), who emphasized how care in nursing homes, especially tasks performed by the aides, has adopted this rationalized approach. This move was initiated by management, because of financial and regulatory pressures. Aides were, because of these pressures, given increasing task workloads, with very specific limits on what they should do (and cannot do) for nursing home residents. The work became highly scheduled, with little opportunity for autonomy or creativity on the part of the workers. The work tasks, which are subsequently charted, counted, and used for performance evaluation and regulatory purposes, are the only behaviors that "count" in terms of the supervisors' views of worker performance (Diamond 1990). This emphasis on instrumental tasks exists despite management ideologies emphasizing caring attention and personalized service to home residents.

Ritzer (1993) emphasized that there are still a few employment settings that have escaped the rationalized task approach of McDonaldization. Board-and-care in small homes may be one setting that has resisted the rationalized task approach that is even coming to characterize medicine (see Ritzer 1993). In these "nonrationalized niches," tasks remain scheduled by the worker, often done in isolation from others, largely free of bureaucratic demands such as required meetings, and tasks are undertaken (to some degree) at the discretion of the worker (Ritzer 1993). Most often, Ritzer suggests, such niches are accessible to those in high-ranking occupation and in situations outside, or as islands within, large-scale organizations (1993).

Small board-and-care homes exemplify many of the characteristics of nonrationalized niches. The operators choose to do this type of work, often after having experienced prior employment in more rationalized health care settings, such as hospitals and nursing homes. Many expressed dissatisfaction at those prior working situations, arguing that they provided better care in the autonomy of their own homes. The work of board-and-care is scheduled at the operator's own pace, with substantial choice (within financial and regulatory constraints) regarding the number and type of residents to accept. The work is often done in isolation from others and is largely free of bureaucratic demands (e.g., meetings, training sessions).

□ OPERATORS OF small board-and-care homes fit well with profiles that have been developed of women working in similar caregiving occupations. Most are mature, and more than would be expected are minorities. Their education is often limited, but they rate their health as good. In the view of the labor force, many of these women would be marginal as workers, unable to command high salaries or work in jobs with security, benefits, and opportunities for advancement. In light of these limitations, choosing to operate a small board-and-care home, including "being your own boss," may hold considerable appeal.

The fact that most had prior experience in other types of health care settings, most notably nursing homes, means that they have tried other employment options and found them somehow wanting. Expressed attitudes regarding nursing homes (mostly negative) and those reflecting their motivations to initiate caring for individuals in their own homes reflect both altruism and a desire to provide better care than many had seen in nursing homes. While financial considerations were a motivator for doing this type of work, they fell far behind the interpersonal aspects of the work in the eyes of the operators. Although money is recognized as necessary to continue providing care, the reasons for entering and remaining in this type of work do not focus on it as the primary factor, since many operators might be able to earn more money (and benefits) elsewhere.

Of course, the possibility remains that the less well motivated operators refused our interviews or that the operators put their best feet forward during the interviews, telling us what they thought we wanted to hear. Stories relayed through the interviews and the quality ratings of the operators tend to refute this latter view, however. Since the interviewers were in most Baltimore homes from four to five separate times over a two-year period (including the resident health evaluation), there were often ample opportunities to observe both casual interactions and the delivery of services. Our overall conclusion for the operators we studied is that most of them provided good care.

The operators of small board-and-care homes in these two studies indicated problematic aspects of their homes' operation but demonstrated low levels of burden. This apparent inconsistency may be related to the marginality of the relationships in the homes, which are neither familial nor professional in nature. Compared with family caregivers, especially those providing assistance to cognitively impaired elders (Birkel and Jones 1989; Chenoweth and Spencer 1986), the board-and-care home operators seemed relatively unburdened. Although our data do not provide proof of why this is so, we suggest that the "detached attachment" enabled by the distinct role relationship between operator and resident and the self-selection of operators are primary explanations. Also related to the latter is the fact that operators can and do select the types of person they care for, a luxury unavailable to families providing care.

There are rules that apply to operators that do not apply to family caregivers, for example, those related to the administration of medication, and as many operators report, dealing with the residents' families can itself be problematic. One operator reported a conflict with a daughter (a nurse) over giving medications, a task that she did "only as a favor" to the family, since she was not licensed and obligated to give medications. The operator finally moved the client when she "could do no more." "When the family doesn't like what I do, I can do no more. But it hurt to have him leave."

A critical issue that remains for future research is that of the limits of care. Operators in these studies indicated some recognition of their own limitations by rejecting certain types of applicants for housing and care, often based on a prior negative experience. But, as we shall see in the next chapter, many homes are caring for exceedingly frail or seriously mentally ill individuals. Cost-containment pressures encourage the removal of these individuals from larger institutions or medical care settings. They require care in some setting, however, and board-and-care homes have taken in many of these deinstitutionalized individuals. Although the operators did not report burden as a significant problem, the question remains as to whether financial pressures prompt them to accept (or to keep) individuals who actually require more care than they can effectively provide (Baggett 1989). Particular concerns have been voiced regarding those requiring considerable supervision, such as individuals with Alzheimer's disease or chronic mental illness (Baggett 1989; Kane, Wilson, and Clemmer 1993). Our pools of operators, with their seemingly high levels of confidence in their abilities to provide care, may be encouraged to take increasingly difficult cases that may exceed their abilities to provide good care for all those in their charge. Discovering mechanisms to manage this dilemma remains for operators with residents whose health is failing or who are disruptive (see chap. 5). Relatively little is known regarding the seriousness and types of impairments found in smaller homes. To address this gap in knowledge, results of the Cleveland resident interviews and the Baltimore health evaluations are described in greater detail in chapter 5.

The operators run their homes in the unmarked, marginal territory between family and formal institution. Many of the problems they encounter (e.g., locating residents, respite, and regulation) derive in a sense from being an underground service-delivery system. They are not organized, case-managed, and funded by a single agency, instead dealing with haphazard and sometimes overlapping interventions from a variety of agencies and groups (Dobkin 1989; Hawes et al. 1993).

The next chapters illuminate further the lives of operators by first describing the characteristics and problems of residents in their homes and then examining in detail the nature of the social context and interactions occurring within the homes between operators and residents. Both chapters elaborate themes introduced here regarding the motivations and actions of operators as unaffiliated providers of care in the irregular economy.

5 □ The Residents

□ ALTHOUGH BOARD-AND-CARE homes serve various populations, some characteristics would be expected to be typical of nearly all of their residents. One such factor is the need for daily assistance or supervision; residents are unable to function independently because of physical and/or mental frailties. In addition, many of the residents lack family members who are able or willing to provide the care that they need (Dittmar et al. 1983; Eckert, Lyon, and Namazi 1990; Mor, Sherwood, and Gutkin 1986; Reichstein and Bergofsky 1983).

If little is known about small board-and-care homes, perhaps even less is known about their clients. Several previous studies (Baggett 1989; Dittmar et al. 1983; Eckert, Lyon, and Namazi 1990; Hawes et al. 1993; McCoin 1983; Mor, Sherwood, and Gutkin 1986; Namazi et al. 1989; Reichstein and Bergofsky 1983; Sherman and Newman 1988), have described the residents of board-and-care-type housing. Although there were notable differences among the facilities studied by these researchers, the similarities among the residents was striking. The findings revealed a mixed population. The first major group consisted of frail older women who were widowed, never married, separated, or divorced. A second major group was composed of deinstitutionalized mental hospital patients, who were predominantly male.

These prior studies have focused on the issues that are primarily of interest to outsiders, such as the appropriateness of placement (Baggett 1989; Dittmar et al. 1983; Hawes et al. 1993; Mor, Sherwood, and Gutkin 1986; Reichstein and Bergofsky 1983), residents' resources for financing board-and-care services (CSSP 1988), and the regulation of the facilities to meet residents' needs (Hawes et al. 1993; Newman 1989). Other authors have explored the issues of quality and residents' rights (Newman 1989; Reisacher 1989). A few studies (Eckert, Lyon, and Namazi 1990; McCoin 1983; Namazi et al. 1989; Sherman and Newman 1988) have taken the insiders' perspective, examining the interpersonal environments of the small board-and-care homes and the residents' satisfaction with their housing and care situations.

This chapter describes the residents of the small board-and-care homes in the Cleveland and Baltimore studies. As noted in chapter 1, residents were interviewed in Cleveland, with a bias in favor of those who were healthier and cognitively intact (see also the appendix). Of considerable importance to caregivers, regulators, and policymakers is the physical and mental health status of these residents. One of the goals of the Baltimore study was to objectively evaluate the health status of a randomly selected sample of older residents to better understand their levels and types of infirmities. In addition to comparing residents in the two locations, comparisons are also made here with other populations, including the general elderly population and people confined to nursing homes. The objective data from the Baltimore study are most useful in providing this information, supplemented by responses from the Cleveland residents. In addition, the chapter explores the movements of residents into and out of the homes and concludes with data from the Cleveland study concerning the residents' satisfaction with the small board-and-care homes.

Data reported in this chapter come from several sources. The Cleveland study reports on 218 residents living in 113 homes meeting our criteria for inclusion in the sample. Although as many as six residents responded to the interview from a single Cleveland board-and-care home, 79.9 percent of the homes had only one or two residents who were interviewed. As noted in chapter 1, approximately one-half of the residents living in the Cleveland homes were not interviewed. In addition to problems due to physical or mental impairments, some residents were screened out by the operators, and others were not in the home at the time of the interviews. A mental status examination, completed during the interview, disqualified an additional twelve residents. These results from the Cleveland study are biased in favor of the less-impaired residents in the homes.

In Baltimore, much of what we know about the residents comes from reports by the operators. Data were collected on up to four residents in the first operator interview, and successive interviews added up to four additional residents as they moved into the homes. In the sample reported here, select information is available on up to 343 residents.

Key health information on the Baltimore residents comes from the health evaluations, conducted by geriatric nurses. Many of the selected residents were not able to participate fully in this evaluation. Of the eighty-five evaluations that were completed, proxies were used for part of the information in some cases ($N = 32$) and for all of the information in others ($N = 16$). In keeping with the earlier chapters, comparisons were frequently made between residents on the basis of the size of the home, the race of the operator, the average fees paid for care, and (in Baltimore) whether the home participated in Project HOME. Given the distinct nature of the Project HOME clientele (dominated by deinstitutionalized, chronically mentally ill persons), special attention is paid to the comparisons on this factor in this chapter.

Who Are Board-and-Care Home Residents?

The characteristics of many residents of board-and-care homes define their marginal status in relation to the larger society. Many of them, as will be seen, fall within age, health, income, and other categories that create this marginality. These characteristics result in a lack of strong ties to the social order, placing them outside the dominant group (Mizruchi 1987).

Demographic Characteristics

Persons who received housing, care, and some amount of protective oversight in small board-and-care homes were most typically women with limited incomes, who were not married, and who were over the age of sixty-five. As the data will continue to reveal, these older female residents were more physically frail than others in the homes and tended to live in larger, white-operated, and higher-fee homes. The remaining dependent adult residents were typically former mental hospital patients who had been deinstitutionalized. They tended to live in smaller board-and-care homes that were operated by African Americans and generally charged lower fees. This follows a pattern identified by other authors (Dittmar et al. 1983; Morrissey 1982; Reichstein and Bergofsky 1983; Sherman and Newman 1988).

Some of the differences between residents in Cleveland and Baltimore may be accounted for by the presence of the Project HOME program (see chap. 1). For example, the resident population in Baltimore differed in terms of age, income, family status, and some of the indicators of health status, from the residents in the Cleveland study. As was the case in prior research, the deinstitutionalized mentally ill, nonetheless, make up a relatively large proportion of the Cleveland residents (Dittmar et al. 1983; Reichstein and Bergofsky 1983).

Table 9 depicts characteristics of the residents in Cleveland and in Baltimore, compared with the general elderly population in 1984 and the population living in nursing homes in 1985 (Senate 1991). Because not all of the board-and-care residents in the studies were over the age of sixty-five, table 9 also includes columns indicating percentages of those residents in that age group, where appropriate. The residents of small board-and-care homes were mostly over the age of sixty-five, with 85.7 percent in Cleveland and 60.2 percent in Baltimore meeting this criterion. Also notable is the fact that among those aged sixty-five or more, nearly one in three of the home residents were above the age of eighty-five, an age when disabilities mount and functionality declines. The presence of more elderly residents in the Cleveland homes may be due to the placement efforts of Project

Table 9

Characteristics of Board-and-Care Home Residents, the U.S. Elderly
Population, and Nursing Home Residents

Characteristic	Cleveland Residents (N = 218)		Baltimore Residents (N = 343)		Living in Community, 1984[a]	Living in Nursing Home, 1985[a]
	All	65+	All	65+		
Age (yr)						
<55	4.1[b,c]	—	18.4[b]	—	—	—
55–64	10.1	—	21.3	—	—	—
65–74	25.2	29.4	21.1	35.0	61.7	16.1
75–84	35.3	41.2	21.6	35.9	30.7	38.6
85+	25.2	29.4	17.5	28.6	7.6	45.3
Sex						
Female	64.2[b]	67.9	64.3[c]	68.0	59.2	74.6
Male	35.8	32.1	35.7	32.0	40.8	25.4
Race						
Black	18.8[b,c,d]	17.1	38.3[b,c,d]	31.1	8.3	6.2
White	81.2	82.9	61.7	68.9	90.4	93.1
Marital status						
Widowed	66.1[c]	74.3	—	—	34.1	67.8
Married	5.0	4.3	11.4	9.2	54.7	12.8
Never married	16.5	11.8	—	—	4.4	13.5
Separated/ divorced	12.4	9.7	—	—	6.3	5.9
Has children	61.5[b,c]	63.1	39.9[b,c]	48.8	81.3	63.1
Receives SSI	11.9[b,c]	9.6	43.3[b,c]	32.2	—	—

Note: Percentages for those living in the community and in nursing homes are for people who are age 65 or over only. The percentages for the Cleveland and Baltimore board-and-care home residents are for all ages, with a deliberate bias toward older residents. Therefore, these are not true comparisons.

[a]*Source*: U.S. Senate Special Committee on Aging, 1991. *Aging in America: Trends and projections*. Washington, D.C., p. 163.

[b]Difference by race of home operator is statistically significant ($p < .05$).

[c]Difference by average fee (low, high) is statistically significant ($p < .05$).

[d]Difference by home size (1–3 vs. 4–8 residents) is statistically significant ($p < .05$).

HOME in Baltimore (see table 10). In both locations, older residents were significantly more likely to live in board-and-care homes having white operators than in those operated by African Americans. In Cleveland, older residents were also significantly more likely to live in higher-fee homes, with nearly three-quarters of the residents in these homes over seventy-five years of age, a figure approaching the 83.9 percent of nursing home residents who were over age seventy-five. As would seem appropri-

Table 10
Baltimore Resident Characteristics
by Facilities' Participation
in Project HOME

	Project HOME Participation	
Characteristic	Yes	No
Age (yr)		
<55	25.9	14.8***
55–64	32.1	16.1
65–74	25.0	19.1
75–84	10.7	27.0
85+	6.3	23.0
Sex		
Female	57.1	67.8*
Male	42.9	32.2
Race		
Black	50.0	32.6**
White	50.0	67.4
Has any family	80.9	91.2*
Has spouse	8.9	12.6
Has children	28.6	45.5**
Receives SSI	66.1	32.2***
Spent time in a mental institution	71.1	37.8**

Note: N = 343.

*Difference between the groups is statistically significant ($p < .05$).

**Difference between the groups is statistically significant ($p < .01$).

***Difference between the groups is statistically significant ($p < .001$).

ate, the residents of board-and-care homes occupied an intermediate position on age, between the elderly who were independent and those who were living in nursing homes. Not surprisingly, this intermediate status of the residents reappears as we look at other characteristics.

The distribution of residents by sex was virtually the same in both Cleveland and Baltimore. A few significant differences in gender were revealed when comparisons were made between homes (see table 9). In Cleveland, women were significantly more likely than men to live in homes operated by white caregivers (68.3 percent vs. 31.7 percent). In comparing residents on the basis of the level of fees paid for care, many more women than men were found in the higher-fee homes in Baltimore (70.6 percent vs. 29.4 percent for men). Confirming their intermediate position, the proportion of board-and-care home residents who were female falls between the figures for community-dwelling elderly and for the population in nursing homes. This is partly a function of the age differences in these various settings, since more women will have survived to the older ages characteristic for nursing home placement (Senate 1991).

Perhaps the most striking contrast revealed by table 9 was the difference in the racial makeup of the resident population. As table 9 shows, there were nearly twice as many African American residents in the Baltimore sample as there were in Cleveland (38.3 percent vs. 18.8 percent). The city of Baltimore has a higher percentage of blacks in its population than does Cleveland (Bureau of the Census 1993), and more of the Baltimore homes were located in the city itself than was the case for Cleveland. Far higher percentages of older African Americans were residing in small board-and-care homes than in either the community or in nursing homes. Blacks may be more likely to live in board-and-care homes than in nursing homes for reasons related to cost, availability of facilities, cultural preference, or other factors (Mindel, Wright, and Starrett 1986).

Within the board-and-care homes in both locations, racial differences appeared across all of the categories we used for comparison (size of home, race of operator, fees paid for services, and participation in Project HOME) (see tables 9 and 10). Significantly more of the residents in the larger homes in Cleveland (88.7 percent) and in Baltimore (76.0 percent) were white. This was also true in the higher-fee homes in Cleveland, in which 70.6 percent of the residents were white, and in Baltimore (97.3 percent white residents). The most telling difference was in the racial distribution of residents by race of the operator. Black residents did not live in homes operated by whites (only 1.8 percent in Cleveland and 0.9 percent in Baltimore), whereas the resident population was more likely to be racially mixed in homes operated by African Americans (25.5 percent in Cleveland and 42.2 percent in Baltimore).

This interracial caregiving may be difficult for residents. Interviewer field notes revealed some of the feelings of a white resident living in a home run by an African American operator in a black neighborhood. The client said, "The neighbors bring me tomatoes. I didn't want nothing to do with the blacks when I came here. But they are good people. They're good to me. We talk, we laugh. I know the baby (operator's grandson) thinks more of me than his own grandmother. I don't think [the grandmother] minds much though."

Nearly all of the operators in Cleveland, regardless of race, said that they would take white residents, while only 70 percent of white operators said that they would take clients who were black, although most apparently did not do so. In the Baltimore study, over 80 percent of white operators had not had any residents of a race different from their own, whereas 73 percent of black operators had cared for residents of another race.

Family Status of Board-and-Care Home Residents

Having family members who are able and willing to care for their dependent kin seems to be an important determinant of who lives in board-and-care homes and who does not (Eckert, Lyon, and Namazi 1990). Mizruchi (1987) identified the lack of important social ties, particularly ties to family, as a key factor contributing to the marginal status of individuals. Findings about the presence of various types of kin for the residents are also detailed in table 9. We first examine the key kinship roles of spouse and child, followed by a description of other kin available to residents.

The Cleveland data provided a breakdown of marital status that showed the highest percentage of residents to be widowed, with a substantial percentage of the widowed housed in higher-fee homes. This mirrors the earlier findings on the higher fees being paid by older female residents, most of whom were widowed. When comparing residents by sex and marital status, female residents were significantly more likely to have been widowed than were their male counterparts, who more often reported never having been married.

Well over half (61.5 percent) of the residents in Cleveland reported one or more children. There were significant variations on this variable by the race of the operator and by the level of fees paid for services. Those living in lower-fee homes or homes operated by an African American were less likely to have children. As table 9 shows, people who were residing in board-and-care homes in Cleveland resembled nursing home residents in terms of marital and parent status. Like nursing home residents, they were twice as likely to be widowed as the elderly living in the community.

In the Baltimore homes, significant differences in the availability of kin emerged when comparing residents in homes that were operated by African Americans or in which fees for services were below average. Significantly fewer of the residents had kin in homes with black operators (83.9 percent vs. 95.7 percent for white operators) and in the lower-fee homes (83.0 percent vs. 93.2 percent for higher-fee homes). Although there were no significant differences among these groups when operators were asked whether the resident had a spouse (most, as expected, did not), significant differences emerged when they were asked about whether the resident had any children (see table 9). In white-operated and higher-fee homes, the residents were more likely to have children (50.0 percent in white-operated homes and 46.3 percent in higher-fee homes), perhaps reflecting cultural and economic differences affecting caregiving choices in families (see table 9).

When comparing the residents in Baltimore by the facility's participation in the Project HOME program (table 10), those who lived in the program homes were significantly less likely to have had children (28.6 percent vs. 45.5 percent) or any other family members (80.9 percent vs. 91.2 percent). Considering the younger ages of this group and their histories of institutionalization, this difference is not surprising (table 10 includes percentages in both groups who reported spending time in a mental institution). Being deinstitutionalized is perhaps doubly marginalizing, through both the stigma of mental illness and the distancing that hospitalization may create from any remaining kin (Germani 1980; Mizruchi 1987).

A higher percentage of the elderly population living in the community (81.3 percent) had living children (see table 9) compared with Cleveland residents (61.5 percent), Baltimore residents (39.9 percent), or residents of nursing homes (63.1 percent). These data support the argument that some residents of pay-for-care environments are there because they lack children to assist them (Soldo 1981).

Although the board-and-care home residents in these studies did not have as many close kin (i.e., spouses and children) as did the other groups profiled in table 9, they did not entirely lack these important social connections (see chap. 6). In Cleveland, operators were asked about the number of residents who were visited by various family members. In the sample, 17.4 percent were visited by their grandchildren, 13.8 percent received visits from their siblings, and other relatives visited 26.1 percent of the residents in the sample. We lack data on whether there were other relatives who were unable or unwilling to make visits to the homes. In Baltimore, where operators provided the information about residents' families, nearly 90 percent of current residents had at least some family. The operators reported that 61.5 percent of their residents had siblings, 30.9 percent had nieces and nephews, some of the residents (14.0 percent) had parents, and a few of them (9.0 percent) had in-laws. About one-tenth of the residents (9.3 percent) had other types of kin including cousins, godchildren, aunts and uncles, grandparents, foster kin, or fictive kin.

Education and Work History

Although limited data were collected regarding the personal history of the residents in Baltimore, Cleveland residents were asked a series of questions including how much school they had completed and what kinds of jobs they had held. More than half (56.4 percent) of the residents interviewed in Cleveland had not completed high school, 27.5 percent graduated from high school, and another 14.7 percent had some college education or a degree. Among those in the population over the age of sixty-five, fewer (45.1 percent) had less than a high school education, and more (33.2 percent) had graduated from high school or gone beyond (21.7 percent) (Taeuber 1992). The low-income status of board-and-care home residents may be largely a function of limited educational attainment.

Despite this limited educational attainment, 14.7 percent of the Cleveland residents claimed to have held jobs as executives, managers, or administrators. An additional 67.4 percent of the Cleveland residents said that they had worked in lower-level clerical or sales jobs or as skilled or unskilled laborers. Another 16.5 percent (all of whom were female) reported having had no occupation. The female residents were more likely to have worked in lower-level jobs (80.0 percent) than were males (60.0 percent). As we shall see, the work histories of many residents of small board-and-care homes left them with very limited financial resources to provide for their needs.

Income

The amount of personal income or program support available to current or potential residents of board-and-care homes determines their range of choices among homes. Some aspects of residents' income have already been discussed in chapter 3. It was not surprising to find that the residents in lower-fee homes in Cleveland were significantly more likely to be receiving SSI (23.4 percent vs. 0.9 percent in higher-fee homes) (see table 9). In both of the locations we studied, African American residents of small board-and-care homes were significantly more likely (27.5 percent in Cleveland and 55.1 percent in Baltimore) than were white residents (7.2 percent, Cleveland, and 20.5 percent, Baltimore) to be receiving SSI. Similarly, more of the residents of homes operated by African Americans were participating in this government program, with its maximum payment of $340 per month at the time the data were collected in Cleveland and $368 to $386 per month when interviews were being conducted in Baltimore. This difference mirrors the general rate of poverty in the United States in 1990, with African Americans over the age of sixty-five (33.8 percent) three times more likely than their white counterparts (10.1 percent) to be poor (Taeuber 1992).

When the Baltimore operators were asked about the sources of income to their residents, comparisons showed that the residents in the smaller homes (three or fewer residents) were significantly more likely to receive SSI (47.6 percent vs. 28.0 percent in larger homes), as were residents in black-operated homes (55.1 percent vs. 20.5 percent in white-operated homes). Surprisingly, there was no significant difference in the proportion of residents in lower- and higher-fee homes who received SSI. This was most likely due to the supplementation from Project HOME for some SSI residents, at that time the highest state supplement in the country (see chaps. 1 and 3). Table 10 shows, not surprisingly, that significantly more Project HOME residents were recipients of SSI (66.1 percent) than were the residents of homes that were not participating in the program (32.2 percent).

One operator's comments to the interviewer addressed the problems created by the low incomes of many residents. One of her residents was able to live more independently, according to her social worker. However, the operator recalled, "I never thought she was ready and I told them. But they thought it was for the best. They didn't give her anything to set her up, no apartment, no furniture, nothing! She got $407 a month. Now where was she going to find an apartment? She moved from relative to relative. But they knew the family drank. She was doomed to fail."

Baltimore operators were also asked whether residents received private pensions. Having had jobs covered by pensions was not characteristic of many board-and-care home residents, because of gender and racial discrimination in employment, interrupted work careers, and histories of mental illness. Few residents in Baltimore (7.9 percent) were receiving funds from a private pension, with residents in white-operated homes and in higher-fee homes predictably more likely to report pension income.

The Health Status of Board-and-Care Home Residents

A central concern of all stakeholders in the board-and-care industry is the appropriateness of placements (i.e., do the environment and services match the level and type of impairment of the resident?). Outsiders, as noted in chapter 1, often question the capacity of board-and-care homes to meet the needs of residents with regard to safety. For example, policymakers, administrators, the media, and the public have all addressed the ability of the residents to escape in the event of fire or other disaster (House 1989). The operators, in turn, wish to set realistic limits for themselves in terms of the ability to meet the needs of individual residents. Some of the health problems typical among board-and-care home residents (e.g., mental illness, dementia) result in problematic behaviors that require management and difficult decisions by the operators regarding relocation. Both the residents and their families seek care and oversight provided in a humane way.

What constitutes an appropriate placement of residents in board-and-care homes, and what can be done to enable homes to better serve their residents? To address these questions, it is essential to have a better understanding of the physical and mental health status of the residents. Unlike more-institutional environments, formal health records are not usually kept in small board-and-care homes. In our two studies, several approaches were taken to build a better picture of resident health status. The health evaluation of older residents in Baltimore was intended to close this gap in knowledge. Although some data on health are available from the Cleveland study, that sample was biased in favor of less-impaired residents, and the interview items were more subjective. Findings in this section, therefore, rely more heavily on data drawn from the operators' interviews and the health evaluations conducted in Baltimore.

Subjective Evaluations of Health Status by Residents

In the Cleveland study, residents were asked to rate their health as poor, fair, good, or excellent. Approximately one-half of the residents rated their health as good, with an additional 12 percent assessing it as excellent. Only 8 percent of residents rated their health as poor, with the remaining 32 percent feeling that it was fair. Significant differences did emerge between groups in this study. The residents of homes operated by African Americans and those paying lower fees rated their health less favorably than did others.

In Baltimore, residents who participated in the health evaluation were asked if health problems stood in the way of doing things. Of those who responded, one-half said not at all, and fewer (27.8 percent) reported that they stood in the way a little. Only one-fifth (20.8 percent) of the residents felt that their health problems stood in their way a great deal. There were no significant differences between our usual comparison groups in the subjective health evaluations in Baltimore.

These findings are interesting in a dependent population and may indicate their mental outlook more than the actual health status of the residents. As Liang (1986) and Stoller (1984) have noted, the relationships among subjective health status, medically determined health status, functional health status, and social-psychological factors are complex. Subjective assessment of physical health has been shown to be closely correlated with psychological well-being (Bradburn 1969).

Functional Health Status of Residents

The residents in Cleveland homes were asked if they needed help in carrying out six activities of daily living (ADLs), including bathing, dressing, grooming, walking, transferring in and out of bed, and toileting. As expected, most of the residents of homes in both locations required some assistance in these areas. The average resident in Cleveland required assistance on only 1.1 of these tasks. There was variation among the tasks, ranging from nearly one-third (31.2 percent) needing help with bathing to only a few (8.7 percent) needing help in toileting (see table 11).

There were significant differences in the ability of residents to carry out these activities in various types of homes. The level of fees being paid made a consistent difference, with more of those in higher-fee homes requiring help with all of the ADLs. Those in the smaller homes and white-operated homes also required more assistance with several ADL tasks.

Baltimore residents (or their proxies) in the health evaluation responded to seven questions on the ADLs (see table 11). This group of residents required more help than did their peers in Cleveland, perhaps as a consequence of the sample bias discussed earlier. The Baltimore residents needed assistance with an average of 2.2 ADLs. Examination of the specific tasks showed that the impairment of the residents in Baltimore was substantially higher on all of them, with the exception of assistance with walking, for which the two samples are virtually identical.

Significant differences in the percentage of residents requiring help with ADLs in the Baltimore homes appeared for the level of fees paid and participation in Project HOME. The residents of higher-fee homes were more often the recipients of assistance in bathing, dressing, and grooming. The younger ages of the Project HOME residents influenced their health status, such that they were significantly less likely to require assistance with bathing, walking, transferring in and out of bed, and toileting. Chapter 3 suggested that operators charged higher fees when residents required more care (i.e., were more impaired). What happens to residents who cannot pay the additional fees if they need more care as their health deteriorates? Are they institutionalized prematurely? As federal and state regulatory and reimbursement policies make it more difficult for people with light-to-moderate care needs to enter nursing homes (Doty 1993), the fate of these impaired residents is in doubt.

The intermediate status of board-and-care home residents (between the home and the long-term care institution) is again revealed when they are compared on ADLs with community-dwelling elderly and with older persons in nursing homes (see table 11). Few older adults living in the community required assistance with any ADLs, but far higher percentages of nursing home residents required assistance (Senate 1991). Using this ADL comparison, the residents in board-and-care homes collectively demonstrated appropriate intermediate placement.

One of the greatest safety concerns expressed about the residents of board-and-care homes is that they be able to escape in the event of fire or

Table 11
Functional Health Status of Board-and-Care Home Residents, the General Elderly Population, and Nursing Home Residents

Characteristic	Cleveland Residents (N = 218)		Baltimore Residents (N = 85)		Living in Community, 1984[a]	Living in Nursing Home, 1985[a]
	All	65+	All	65+		
Activities of daily living, needs help with:						
Bathing	31.2[b]	33.7	51.8[b,c]	58.2	6.0	91.0
Eating	—	—	21.7	20.0	1.1	40.3
Dressing	19.3[b,d]	20.3	42.2[b]	49.1	4.3	77.6
Grooming	14.2[b,d,e]	16.0	42.7[b]	46.3	—	—
Walking	21.1[b]	23.0	22.9[c]	32.7	—	—
Transferring	11.9[b,e]	12.8	18.1[c]	25.5	2.8	62.6
Toileting	8.7[b,e]	9.1	23.5[c]	29.6	2.2	63.2
Taking medications	30.3	29.9	75.3	72.3	—	—
Not able to exit facility independently	—	—	41.0[c]	49.1	—	—

Note: Percentages for those living in the community and in nursing homes are for people who are age 65 or over only. The percentages for the Cleveland and Baltimore board-and-care home residents are for all ages, with a deliberate bias toward older residents. Therefore, these are not true comparisons.

[a]Source: U.S. Senate Special Committee on Aging, 1991. *Aging in America: Trends and projections.* Washington, D.C., p. 163.

[b]Difference by average fee (low, high) is statistically significant ($p < .05$).

[c]Difference by program participation (Project HOME, non-Project HOME) is statistically significant ($p < .05$).

[d]Difference by home size (1–3 vs. 4–8 residents) is statistically significant ($p < .05$).

[e]Difference by race of home operator is statistically significant ($p < .05$).

other disaster. One question in the health evaluation of Baltimore residents concerned the ability of the subject to exit the facility independently. As table 11 shows, in this randomly selected sample of older residents of small board-and-care homes, 41 percent were judged *not* able to meet this standard, subjecting them to greater risk in the event of fire. In the minds of many outsiders, this strongly suggests inappropriate placement of these individuals. Only when comparing homes by program affiliation did a statistically significant difference occur, with the rather (physically) healthy residents in Project HOME facilities more likely to be able to exit the facility independently.

According to an interviewer's field notes, one operator said that occasionally she held fire drills as a way of preparing her clients for an emergency, especially if she was away from the home. "She stressed to her clients that death may be around the corner for each of them and they must live their lives fully and always be prepared for the unexpected."

Indicators of Health Problems in Baltimore Residents

Table 12 presents percentages of residents from the Baltimore study's health evaluation with symptoms of physical health problems. The percentages reflect those who said that they had the symptom or health status indicator at least sometimes.

Many of the most common problems, such as difficulty moving joints (38.8 percent), joint pain (44.7 percent), dry skin and rashes (41.2 percent), corns and bunions (35.7 percent), and problems with gums and teeth (40.0 percent; 32 percent had dentures), were those generally noted in the frail elderly population. Between one-fifth and one-third of the residents reported indicators of other, more serious, health problems.

Troubles with respiration included shortness of breath (31.8 percent), frequent cough (22.4 percent), and sleeping propped up by pillows to ease breathing (22.6 percent). About one-third of the residents smoked cigarettes, with 59 percent of smokers consuming more than one pack a day. Among the cardiovascular problems, swollen ankles and legs (28.2 percent), numbness or tingling in parts of the body (20.0 percent), dizziness (25.9 percent), fainting (18.8 percent), and having experienced pain in the chest (21.2 percent) were all fairly common.

Significant percentages of the residents also had problems affecting gastrointestinal and genitourinary systems. Twenty percent had difficulty chewing or swallowing, perhaps because of problems with gums or teeth. Nearly as many (18.8 percent) had digestive problems, indicated by gas or belching, indigestion, queasiness, diarrhea, or gastric ulcers; and 34.1 percent required a special diet. The specific special diets mentioned were low-

Table 12

Health Indicators in Baltimore Residents

System/Indicator	Percentage ($N = 85$)
Musculoskeletal/skin	
Couldn't move joints as should	38.8
Pain in joints	44.7[a]
Skin problems	41.2
Pressure areas	7.2[a]
Corns, bunions	35.7
Respiratory	
Ever short of breath	31.8
Frequent cough	22.4
Sleeps propped up to ease breathing	22.6
Smokes cigarettes	32.9[a]
Cardiovascular	
Swollen ankles and legs	28.2[a]
Numbness or tingling	20.0[b]
Dizziness	25.9
Has fainted	18.8
Has had chest pain	21.2
Gastrointestinal	
Problems with gums, teeth	40.0[b]
Difficulty chewing or swallowing	20.0
Constipation	34.1
Diarrhea	29.4
Stomach problems	18.8[a,b]
Needs special diet	34.1[c]
Genitourinary	
Frequent urination	35.9
Has had accident getting to toilet	17.7
Neurological	
Has had seizure	16.5
Has had stroke	20.0[a,b]
Vision problems	23.8
Weakness in muscles	18.4

Note: Responses were based on resident or proxy report (37 residents answered questions for themselves, 32 participated with another person, usually the operator, 16 required total assistance in responding) or nurse/interviewer observation.

[a]Difference by program participation (Project HOME, non–Project HOME) is statistically significant ($p < .05$).

[b]Difference by race of home operator is statistically significant ($p < .05$).

[c]Difference by home size (1–3 vs. 4–8 residents) is statistically significant ($p < .05$).

salt, diabetic, multiple (more than one limitation), and pureed food. Constipation (34.1 percent) and diarrhea (29.4 percent) were both specified as problems for substantial minorities of the residents evaluated.

Having difficulty getting to the toilet in time (17.7 percent) was not uncommon, with over one-third (37 percent) of the residents in this group reporting it as a frequent problem. As noted in chapter 4, incontinence of bowel or of bladder were conditions identified by many operators as not acceptable in potential residents. Many residents also developed problems with continence while living in the board-and-care homes. An interviewer reported, "[A]s time has passed, I have noticed an odor of urine coming from [this resident's] room. This is consistent with what the operator has told me about the client's increasing difficulties with incontinence." In another instance, the interviewer reported, "Being clean and dry is *very* important to this operator. What was particularly troublesome for the operator was not that the client had been confused, disruptive, or incontinent, but that the operator had no way of controlling the client to keep her safe and clean." This client was later placed in a nursing home.

Some of the operators and residents managed problems with continence in several ways, including using adult diapers and undergarments (16 percent of the residents use them), taking the resident to the toilet every two hours or reminding them to go, keeping a bedpan nearby, using special toilets, and avoiding certain kinds of food and drink. Frequent urination was also identified as a problem for 35.9 percent of the residents, as were pain while urinating (2.9 percent), being unable to urinate (13.6 percent), or having a problem knowing when they have to empty the bladder (24.3 percent). A small number of residents had colostomies (2.0 percent), and a few had catheters (5.0 percent), both of which require some training and skill on the part of the operator to prevent infection.

The most commonly identified neurological problems were seizures (16.5 percent), strokes (20.0 percent), and weakness in muscles (ataxia) (18.4 percent). Vision problems were identified for 23.8 percent of the residents, and 37 percent of them wore glasses. A few of the residents (3.0 percent) used a hearing aid.

To assist residents with disabilities, some homes had special equipment. The equipment included hospital beds in 5.8 percent of the homes, and bath chairs, geriatric chairs, tub rails, gastronomy tubes, and devices to prevent or relieve decubitus ulcers, each present in 1.0 percent of the homes. As previously mentioned, a few of the residents had colostomies or catheters, and some used wheelchairs (10 percent) or walkers (6 percent) because they had difficulty ambulating. Some of this equipment, although it may increasingly be found in private residences (Glazer 1990), is associated with more-skilled medical care that usually requires licensure by the state. The question remains as to whether the board-and-care home opera-tors have the training, skill, and knowledge to care for some of these more seriously impaired residents.

Interviewer notes are again revealing. "The client is on oxygen in the home. A home health nurse came to visit with the client and reported to the operator that she felt the client was making progress. From the conver-sation, it seemed the client suffered from occasional confusion and the operator had difficulty keeping the nasal cannula on the client during the day." One operator put a hospital bed in her dining room for seven months while a client awaited a nursing home slot. Apparently this client was totally bed-bound.

There were several significant differences in these health indicators, on the basis of participation in Project HOME, the race of the operator, and the size of the home. With the exception of smoking cigarettes, a risk factor rather than a symptom, residents in homes participating in the Project HOME program less commonly had joint pain, swelling of the legs and ankles, stomach problems, and a history of stroke, among others. More of the residents in white-operated homes experienced numbness and tin-gling of the extremities, stomach problems, and prior stroke. The residents in homes operated by an African American, by contrast, were significantly more likely to report problems with their gums and teeth. In addition, significantly more residents in smaller homes required special diets. There were no significant differences in any of these health indicators when residents were compared by the average fees paid for services.

Medications

Ongoing professional monitoring and appropriate administration of the medications taken by board-and-care home residents have been issues of concern to policymakers and regulators (Avorn et al. 1989; Blake 1987). Most operators of small homes supervise the residents who are taking medications, but they are not legally permitted to administer them. As was discussed in chapter 4, this indicates the operator's marginal status; she is neither kin nor professional. In family homes, caregiving kin can adminis-ter medications to children or dependent adults without legal interference, as can approved professionals or paraprofessionals in more formal set-tings, such as nursing homes.

An interviewer's field notes reported a case that addresses some of the problems that the operator's marginal status can engender. A female resi-dent was unable to live independently because she was falling frequently. The operator questioned whether the resident needed the medications she was taking for pain and sleeping problems. This operator filled the sleeping capsules with coffee creamer and substituted baby aspirin for the pre-scription pain pill. The resident subsequently improved to the point that her family decided she could return to her apartment. After she moved, the resident's daughter returned to the original medication regimen, and her mother's health deteriorated again. The operator said, "I told her (the daughter) that she didn't need all those medicines. But she said, 'The doctor ordered her to have them.' 'But that's because she's always com-plaining,' I told her." The client moved back into the operator's home, where she stayed until her death.

The difference between residents in Cleveland and Baltimore is also signaled by the amount of assistance required in taking medications. Over-all, fewer than one-third of the Cleveland residents (30.3 percent) reported needing assistance with taking medications, while over three-quarters (75.3 percent) of the Baltimore residents needed some help with this activ-ity (see table 11). As we will see, disruptive behaviors exhibited by resi-dents were sometimes related to problems with medications. According to one operator, "[The mentally unstable] have to be watched all the time. Sometimes they don't take their medicine, and you can't control them. It can become very difficult."

In a conversation with a psychiatrist, another operator was told that her resident would be fine once they adjusted her medication. The operator discovered that the client had not been taking her pills. She said, "But I told the doctor that we gave her medicine three times a day. [We] laid it out on the table. She took it and swallowed it. He said that she would just squirrel it in her mouth, hold it in her cheeks and pretend that she swallowed it. So I said to him, 'Well then, how am I ever going to know?' "

In another case, the operator learned that the medications of a resident demonstrating behavioral problems had not been evaluated in a few years. When she arranged for the medications to be adjusted, the resident's be-havior returned to normal. However, for some residents, medications pre-sent no problems. One nurse evaluator's notes report that one resident being evaluated took care of her own medications. She ordered them and asked the operator to take her to the pharmacy when she needed refills. She appeared to be very knowledgeable about her own health.

Data from the health evaluations of residents in Baltimore provide fur-ther detail on the medications used by board-and-care home residents. Overall, 85.9 percent of the residents evaluated were taking one or more prescription drugs. Among these older residents, the average number of prescription medications being taken was three. Although there were no significant variations in the number of medications taken by most of our comparison variables, white residents took significantly more medications than did African American residents.

Because there was such a high percentage of residents with a history of mental illness, it was not surprising that antipsychotic medications were among those most commonly taken, as well as antiseizure and central nervous system drugs. Well over one-half of the residents (59.0 percent) took such medications, with significantly more of those, as we would expect, living in homes affiliated with Project HOME. Other medications most often mentioned were potassium (14.5 percent), antihypertensives (15.7 percent), diuretics (20.5 percent), nitrates (13.2 percent), vitamins (9.6 percent), and bronchial relaxers (10.8 percent). In addition, many of the residents (44.7 percent) took over-the-counter medications including aspirin, antacids, and laxatives.

Further probes revealed few problems with the use of medications. Eight percent of the residents had run out of their medicine at some time, 5 percent had experienced trouble getting a doctor to renew a prescription, and only 3 percent reported having had trouble affording the drugs that were prescribed for them.

Mental Health and Cognitive Impairment among Home Residents

The deinstitutionalization movement has played a key role in the growth of the board-and-care industry (Blake 1987; Donahue and Oriol 1981). In both the Cleveland and the Baltimore studies, residents (or their proxies in Baltimore) were asked whether they had ever spent time in a mental hospital. There was no systematic variation in these percentages according to the size of the home, the race of the operator, or the level of fees paid for services in either location.

Many more of the Baltimore residents (53.0 percent) had been in mental hospitals than was true of the Cleveland residents (21.1 percent). The effect of Project HOME in Baltimore is part of this difference, since 61.4 percent of residents in participating homes reported prior mental hospitalization, compared with 38.6 percent of those in nonparticipating homes (see table 10). Even without Project HOME, however, the percentage reported to have been in a mental institution is higher in Baltimore, a difference that may be attributable to the sample bias toward healthier individuals in Cleveland.

As the age of the residents increases, problems associated with mental illness may be augmented by cognitive impairment from Alzheimer's disease or other dementing illness. To address the cognitive status of all of the residents, the Baltimore health evaluation included a modified Mini-Mental Status Examination (MMSE) (Folstein, Folstein, and McHugh 1975). On a thirty-point scale, nearly one-third (31.3 percent) of the evaluated residents scored less than sixteen points, indicating cognitive impairment. Since lower scores on the MMSE are associated with lower socioeconomic status and education (Frisoni et al. 1993; Launer et al. 1993), the lower scores of many residents may reflect these factors. Fewer of the residents in Project HOME affiliates had scores on this measure indicating impairment (21.1 percent vs. 40.0 percent, difference not significant), because this instrument assesses cognitive impairment, not mental illness.

Disruptive Behaviors

In recent studies of both board-and-care and assisted living facilities, the operators described the most difficult tenants as those with mental health or emotional problems, rather than those requiring the most physical care (Hawes et al. 1993; Kane, Wilson, and Clemmer 1993). As was discussed in chapter 4, the operators in both locations were aware of the types of residents they were unwilling to take into their homes. These restrictions concentrated on those residents who exhibited difficult behaviors, such as heavy drinking, wandering, drug use, and incontinence. An unexpected result emerging from our studies was the degree to which disruptive behaviors of residents played a role in the stress of operators and the removal of these troublesome residents from the homes.

Much of the discussion about the residents in the interviewers' field notes involved those who displayed disruptive behaviors. "The client with Alzheimer's is becoming progressively worse. The operator stated that she was unsure how long she would be able to keep her in the home. The client needs constant supervision. She rips her hose, stands up and urinates on the carpet, takes her underwear off, etc. 'You'd be surprised how fast these little old people move. I can't take my eyes off her one minute!' " That resident had been moved to a nursing home by the time of the next interview.

Another operator described problems with inappropriate sexual behavior. "One male client made advances on her and another sexually molested her four-month-old daughter." In another home, a male resident was described by his home's operator as very difficult to get along with, often disrupting the home. The resident suffered from spastic muscular movements, which frequently caused him to break things or damage the home. Since the client could not get to the bathroom on time, he carried a metal can for his urine. Many times the urine would spill on the rugs, the furniture, and the walls. This upset both him and the other clients, sometimes resulting in confrontations.

The problems presented by residents with dementia were often discussed by the operators. One resident, apparently suffering from Alzheimer's disease, did such things as wash her clothes by hand at odd hours of the morning and night. She hung them up dripping wet and played the radio loudly, disturbing the other residents. When the operator told her not to do this, the client informed her that she could do whatever she wanted, whenever she wanted. On another occasion in the same home, "her other client screamed, and she turned to find the new client getting ready to hit her." In another home, during the night before the interviewer's visit a resident with Alzheimer's disease had been awake since 2:00 A.M., trying to climb out of his bed. Both he and the operator were exhausted from the night-long confrontation.

Finally, an operator discussed her feelings about a client who had been difficult at times. "The operator told me earlier in the interview that B.'s mental capacity was deteriorating. She had been told to seek nursing home placement for her, because of the amount of supervision needed in her care. However, the operator stated she was determined to keep her for as long as possible. She did not feel B. would survive long in a nursing home setting and, based on her experiences as an aide in this type of facility, she also felt the client would be hurt and abused. 'She's 87 years old and she deserves some sort of good life. You know if she goes to a nursing home, she's gonna die. I've worked in enough of them to know that. They've got three shifts . . . you don't know if they're getting treated well.' This particular concern about treatment was due to the client's tendency to spark arguments with other clients. 'B. . . . has quite a mouth, if you know what I mean.' "

Moving in and out of Board-and-Care Homes

People move into board-and-care homes because they cannot live independently, and they are seeking a supportive residential care environment. They remain in the homes for varying lengths of time; the duration of stay depending on many factors. In addition to learning about where board-and-care residents had lived prior to moving into the facilities and how long they had lived there, the research sought to determine where residents went when they left a home, why they left, and how the decision to depart was made. The residents in Cleveland were asked where they had been living prior to moving into the board-and-care home and how long they had been in the home. The Cleveland operators reported on the places where former residents had gone upon their departures. In Baltimore, operators reported this information about the residents profiled, and an additional series of questions asked them about the circumstances of the resident who had most recently left the home.

Previous Residence

Nearly one-half of the residents in Cleveland had lived in their own homes before relocation to the board-and-care home (see fig. 19). Another 20.6 percent had lived in another residential care home, 16.1 percent had resided with a relative or friend, and 8.7 percent had entered from a nursing home. There was a significant difference between lower- and higher-fee homes, with residents in higher-fee homes more likely to have moved from their own homes, and those in lower-fee homes more likely to have lived in a nursing home or in a relative's home prior to the board-and-care home.

Over one-quarter (26.2 percent) of the resident population in the homes we studied in Baltimore had been living in another board-and-care home previously, and 19.8 percent had been in a mental institution. Smaller percentages of Baltimore residents had moved from a hospital to the home (14.6 percent), had been in their own home (14.5 percent), or had lived with a relative or a friend (11.7 percent). The difference between the two locations, with more residents in Baltimore having moved from another board-and-care home or from a mental institution, indicate the placement efforts of Project HOME in Maryland.

Although only a few of the residents in Baltimore had moved into the board-and-care home from living on the street or in a shelter (see fig. 19), this is likely to happen in urban areas. Interviewer field notes reveal the poignancy of one encounter. The operator discussed a client she took in who had been living on the streets. "He was a young man. He couldn't walk, he had something wrong with his feet. He had to use crutches. He

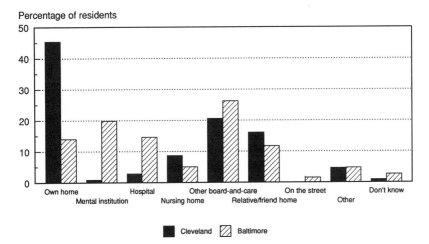

Fig. 19. Previous Residence of Board-and-Care Home Clients

had nowhere to go. It was winter, snow on the ground. He needed someone." In another home, the operator described how one resident came to live there. As the operator was preparing the home for occupancy, she noticed that an elderly woman frequented the park across the street. She went to the woman and asked if she wanted to live with her. The woman stated that she had been watching her fix up the home and was hoping to have a nice place like that to live in. "She moved in carrying all that she owned in her shopping cart," the operator recalled. The woman had been with the operator ever since that day, and the operator was paid $200 a month to care for her. "That's all she has."

Length of Stay

As figure 20 illustrates, nearly two-thirds (61.9 percent) of the residents in Cleveland reported having been in the current home for less than one year, with an additional one-third (33.5 percent) having been there between one and five years. There was little difference in the lengths of stay for residents when comparing by size of the home or by the fees paid for services. Homes with white operators had significantly higher lengths of stay. The same operator described above, who housed a bed-bound resident in her dining room for seven months, had another client who had lived with her for sixteen years and a third for eleven years.

As figure 20 shows, the residents in Baltimore had lived in their current

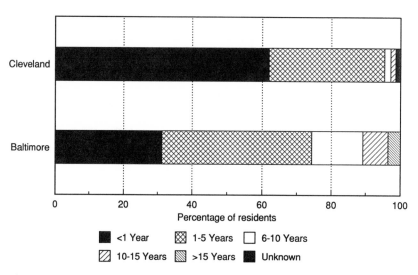

Fig. 20. Length of Stay of Residents of Board-and-Care Homes

board-and-care homes longer than had their counterparts in Cleveland. Nearly one-third (31.2 percent) had been in the home for less than a year, and 43.1 percent had been there for one to five years. In contrast to the lower figures for Cleveland, 14.9 percent of Baltimore residents were in place for six to ten years, and a striking 10.8 percent had lived in the home for more than ten years. One resident had been in the same home for a remarkable twenty-five years! The median length of stay for the residents who were in the Baltimore homes at the time of the first interview ($N = 246$) was forty-two months (3.5 years).

There was a significant difference in length of stay when comparing the Baltimore residents by size of the home, with those in homes of four to eight residents more likely to have resided there longer. However, the smaller board-and-care homes housed the few residents (4.5 percent) who had lived in the board-and-care homes the longest (fifteen years or more). There was also a significant difference based on the average fee, with residents in lower-fee homes generally more likely to have been there longer. Perhaps residents can afford to remain longer in the homes that cost less *because* they cost less. Alternatively, this may be an artifact of the greater physical frailty among the residents of higher-fee homes, who more often face institutionalization or death. A final factor in this difference may have to do with disruptive behaviors. Project HOME subsidies push their participating homes into the higher-fee category. The disruptive behaviors of some clients in this program, as described earlier, may reduce the average length of stay, as the program relocates them, seeking appropriate placements.

Resident Departures: Destinations and Causes

The majority (71.9 percent) of operators in Cleveland, who had experienced one or more client departures, were asked whether they had residents leave to a list of eight possible destinations. Over half said that at least one of their former residents had gone to a hospital (60.4 percent), had died (59 percent), or had gone to a nursing home (56.8 percent). An additional one in three (33.8 percent) said that former residents had relocated to the psychiatric department of a hospital or to a psychiatric hospital. Not all departures were related to worsening condition of the resident. Some operators had clients who had gone back to their own homes (34.5 percent), to live with family members (28.8 percent), or to another board-and-care home (33.8 percent).

To better understand issues leading to operator-initiated departures, the Baltimore operators were asked if they had ever considered removing any of their current residents and, if so, their reasons. The operators had

considered this option for 69 of the residents profiled (20.1 percent). There
were no significant differences on the basis of the size of the home, the race
of the operator, or the average fees paid for services. Among the reasons
offered by operators for considering removal of the resident, 66.7 percent
concerned a behavioral problem, including violent or combative behavior.
The second most common reason (20.3 percent of these responses) was
that the client was too demanding. In fewer of the cases (13.0 percent)
deterioration in the resident's health was given as the reason for considering relocation, with incontinence (11.6 percent) another key reason. A few
operators also mentioned personality conflicts with residents (5.8 percent), the resident's dirtiness (1.4 percent), problems with payment for
services (4.3 percent), or problems with the resident's family (1.4 percent)
as reasons for considering removal of their current residents from the
board-and-care homes.

In a separate question, the operators in Baltimore were asked about the
most important reasons clients had left their homes permanently. In contrast to the problems mentioned above, the most frequently reported reason was death of the resident, with decline in health being second, and
problems with behavior ranking third. It appears that operators considered removal because of behavioral problems more than they followed
through on it.

Interviewer field notes reported on some of the residents' moves out of
the board-and-care homes. "I was surprised to find that the only elderly
client in this home has left and been placed in a nursing home. Apparently
she suffered with increased problems from a rectal prolapse. Attempts had
been made to suture it in place but failed and no other surgical procedures
were possible because of the client's physical and mental health conditions. As a result, she became increasingly incontinent and there was
worry that she would cause further damage to the prolapse. The client's
roommate was disrupted by the odor and incontinence of the client. The
move was determined to be in the best interests of the client and the
home."

Another operator said that she had requested that one client be moved
out of the home because of a progressively worsening problem of incontinence. "They are trying to make me feel guilty because she will have to go
to a nursing home. They know how bad I felt about having T. go there, but I
just couldn't do [it] anymore."

Baltimore Residents Who Left Most Recently

To gain further detail on the circumstances of residents' departures from
small board-and-care homes, operators in Baltimore were asked a series of
questions about the resident who had most recently left, excluding those

who died. In this series of questions, operators also described the length of stay for those who left, reasons for their departures, and their destinations. As the findings in table 13 show, there were two groups of leavers, younger males from the smaller board-and-care homes and older women from the larger homes. Although younger residents were only 18.4 percent of the total, they constituted nearly one-third (32.1 percent) of those recently departing the homes. Similarly, more males left than would have been expected on the basis of their representation in the homes. Those who left were heavily concentrated among the shorter stays, with the great majority (85.2 percent) having been in the home less than five years. Mirroring earlier findings, the most common reason for departure was problematic behavior, followed by a resident's decision and need for more care. The most common destinations were another board and care home (29.6 percent) or living in the community, often with a friend or relative (25.9 percent).

There were few significant differences among homes, using our usual comparison groups, perhaps because of the small number of departures described ($N = 69$). Significant differences emerged for the age of departing residents by home size and by race of the operator. Older residents (over seventy-five years of age) were significantly more likely to have departed from larger and white-operated homes, as would be expected by their concentration in such homes. Similarly, those departing from Project HOME affiliates were younger than those from nonparticipating homes.

When comparing the sex of those who had most recently departed from the homes, only the level of fees paid for board-and-care services was statistically significant. More males (57.6 percent were male) left the lower-fee homes, while in the higher-fee homes, the largest percentage of females (68.8 percent were female) had departed. This difference was expected, since most of the residents who lived in the higher-fee homes were older women.

There were also significant differences in the reasons for leaving the home and the destination of the former resident by whether or not it was a Project HOME participant. The highest percentage (44.4) of the Project HOME residents left because their behavior was a problem, followed by the resident's decision to leave in 25.9 percent of the cases; residents left nonprogram homes because they needed more care (27.0 percent) or the resident decided to leave (21.6 percent). The Project HOME residents went to a mental hospital (25.0 percent) or to another board-and-care home (28.6 percent). Their counterparts in the homes that were not part of the program went to a nursing home (35.9 percent), a family member's home, friend's home, or their own home (28.2 percent), and 23.1 percent of them went to another board-and-care home.

Although many other differences did not reach statistically significant

Table 13
Baltimore Operator Reports of Residents
Who Left Most Recently

Characteristic	Percentage ($N = 69$)
Age (yr)	
<55	32.1[a,b,c]
55–64	17.9
65–74	17.9
75–84	12.5
85+	19.6
Sex	
Female	55.6[d]
Male	44.4
How long resided in the home (yr)	
<1	38.9
1–5	46.3
6–10	11.1
>10	3.7
Reason for leaving	
Behavior a problem	30.8[c]
Resident decided	25.0
Needed more care	19.2
Moved by social worker	9.6
Other reason given	9.6
Family available to care	5.8
Where resident went	
Other board-and-care home	29.6[c]
Family/friend/own home	25.9
Nursing home	18.5
Mental hospital	14.8
Hospital	3.7
Other	3.7
Missing	3.7

[a]Difference by home size (1–3 vs. 4–8 residents) is statistically significant ($p < .05$).

[b]Difference by race of home operator is statistically significant ($p < .05$).

[c]Difference by program participation (Project HOME, non–Project HOME) is statistically significant ($p < .05$).

[d]Difference by average fee (low, high) is statistically significant ($p < .05$).

levels, some of them were quite interesting. For example, one-third of leavers in larger homes needed more care, whereas nearly this number (30.8 percent) left the smaller homes because of behavior problems. Problems with behavior also accounted for one-third of the departures from homes operated by whites and from those charging higher fees. Only in the larger homes was problematic behavior an infrequently mentioned reason for the departure of residents (8.3 percent). Across comparison groups, between 16.7 percent and 26.3 percent of residents were reported by operators to have left because they decided to do so.

One operator described a resident who moved back into his own apartment. The man had Parkinson's disease; he had become very frail and had been hospitalized. The operator had been asked by the hospital to take him temporarily. He stayed for several months, and the operator had become quite attached to him. According to the interviewer, "At one point, the gentleman told the operator that he felt he was well enough to return to his home and the operator agreed with his decision. At that point she helped him set up services (find someone to come in regularly). She states that he left, and she calls every other week to check to see if he needs anything and see how he is doing."

Another operator's story portrays the difficult decisions that are made concerning the departures of residents. An elderly aunt of the operator had been living in the home for several years and had moved to a nursing home to recuperate from a fall. Because the state did not recognize the aunt as family, the operator was told that she could not return to his home unless he gave up one of his clients. Since his aunt had already been moved, he decided to find a placement for her outside of the board-and-care home, instead of choosing which client must leave.

Resident Satisfaction in Board-and-Care Homes

The measurement of resident satisfaction is problematic. First, measurement may require expensive and intensive data collection strategies, which are often deemed impractical by researchers or regulators (Lyon 1993). Second, reliance on self-reports of satisfaction or outcomes by residents presents problems of validity, because of the cognitive impairments and mental illness that characterize many who are housed in residential care facilities (Lyon 1993).

Reisacher (1989) has based her definition of quality in board-and-care homes on standards for residents' rights. These may include the right to privacy; to freedom from abuse, neglect, and exploitation; to voice grievances; and to engage in religious practices and social activities of the resident's choice (Reisacher 1989). Regulatory standards have been established (Stone 1991, 1) to "enhance the dignity, independence, individuality, privacy, choice, and decisionmaking ability of the resident." These aspects of quality may be seen as being key to resident satisfaction. They are not only difficult to measure, but seldom have residents in board-and-care homes been queried on these factors. One outcome measure that has been used in these settings, acknowledging its limitations, is resident satisfaction with the environment (Namazi et al. 1989).

In the Cleveland study, residents were asked a number of questions reflecting their satisfaction with the physical and social environment of the small board-and-care homes. A prior analysis of the Cleveland data (Namazi et al. 1989) found that 27 percent of the residents in Cleveland demonstrated high scores on the Bradburn Affect Balance Scale; 58 percent of the residents had scores reflecting moderate well-being, and only 15 percent had low scores. Using a regression model, it was shown that 31 percent of the variation in well-being was explained by physical and social factors in the board-and-care environment. These factors included the residents' comfort with the home, their comfort with other residents, the quality of interactions with others, the availability of special diets, the cost of the services, and sharing of meals with the operator. Other factors, including presence of steps in the home, the level of noise, and the proximity of public transportation, explained only a small part of the psychological well-being of residents.

The Cleveland residents were asked directly if they liked living in the board-and-care home. Over one-quarter of them (28.4 percent) said that they liked it very much, 64.7 percent said that they often or sometimes liked it, and only 5 percent of the residents did not like living in the board-and-care home at all. When asked if they felt comfortable in the facility, 88.1 percent answered in the affirmative. The reason given most frequently by those who did not feel comfortable (7 of a possible 218 residents) was that the facility was not like a home. Those who were comfortable said that the people that they lived with were friendly, kind, helpful, trustworthy, and reliable (see chap. 6) and that the physical environment was acceptable.

Additional questions in the interview with Cleveland-area board-and-care home residents dealt with some of the factors in the environment that contributed to their satisfaction. Most of the residents (83.5 percent) felt that the food was good (14.2 percent said fair, and only 1.8 percent rated the food poor). Almost all residents (98.2 percent) said that they got enough food to eat, although snacks were only provided to 24.3 percent of them. Only 4.6 percent of the residents complained that the temperature in the home was not comfortable. When asked if the board-and-care home cost more than it was worth, 67.9 percent said that it did not, because they received good care, they were not in an institution, the food was good, or they got what they paid for. The 18.8 percent of residents who were unhappy about the cost of their board-and-care home felt that the cost was too high or that they did not get enough care.

Residents should feel safe in the board-and-care home (Reisacher 1989), and most of them (96.8 percent) said that they did; 90.8 percent felt safe in the neighborhood. None of the residents in the Cleveland sample had faced a problem that threatened their safety in the community. Space and privacy are also assumed to be important to residents (Stone 1991). Nearly all of those responding in the interviews (94.5 percent) said they had enough privacy in the home. The same proportion said that they had enough space (94.5 percent).

Finally, an issue of importance is resident choice and autonomy (Reisacher 1989; Stone 1991). Residents were asked if there were too many rules in the home. Only one person felt that there were too many rules, and almost all of the residents (93.1 percent), as reported in chapter 2, said that there were not any rules they did not like.

According to their responses, the board-and-care home residents who were interviewed in the Cleveland study appeared to be satisfied with many aspects of their care, although there were restrictions on their behavior that many of us would find unacceptable. This may reflect a "fit" between the resident's needs for security, interaction with others, comfort, and care and the ability of the board-and-care home to meet those needs (Eckert, Lyon, and Namazi 1990; Kahana 1982).

□ OUR DATA on the demographic traits and health status of the residents of small board-and-care homes show them to hold an appropriate, intermediate position between those living in the community and people who are housed in nursing homes. The oldest residents were most likely to be women, while younger residents, whose backgrounds often included having spent time in a mental institution, were more likely to be men. Board-and-care home residents were also more likely to be African American than were populations living in the community or in nursing homes. Many of them did not have close kin available to provide the extensive support and personal care required by them, on an ongoing basis.

The physical and mental frailties in these groups created dependencies that resulted in their placement in board-and-care facilities. Some of these frailties were relatively severe and required knowledge and skills (e.g., catheter care) beyond the expertise of the operators of some board-and-care homes. As Glazer (1990) pointed out, however, similarly skilled types of care are now routinely expected of family members with little training and less experience than the home operators we studied.

Our original interest in board-and-care homes developed through gerontology. Beyond the substantial numbers of elderly persons housed there, we found, in confirmation of other studies, a large number of chronically mentally ill residents. Although the presence of Project HOME altered the Baltimore sample, Cleveland homes also housed a remarkably high (about 20 percent) proportion of people who had spent some time in a mental institution. Although not all faced chronic mental illness, many in this group required management of medications and behavior. The interviews in Cleveland, using a sample biased toward higher-functioning residents, nonetheless revealed cognitive impairment in some of the residents. The Baltimore data were more explicit in demonstrating that a high proportion of residents were cognitively impaired.

Residents were more likely to have arrived in the studied homes from another board-and-care facility, a hospital, or a mental institution than from their own homes. The length of time that residents stayed varied. Some residents had been there for a long time and had become part of the family, according to operator reports. Others, especially those with disruptive behaviors, had short stays as they moved from home to home, attempting to find an appropriate environment and care. When residents left the board-and-care homes, it was because they required more care because of physical deterioration, because their behavior had become unmanageable, or they died.

The interviewers' field notes revealed that the disruptive behavior displayed by residents was a frequent topic of the informal conversations during the interview process. Some of this behavior came from residents who had been identified as mentally ill. Much of the disruptive behavior that distressed the operators and led to removals from the homes was from residents diagnosed with Alzheimer's disease. Since the number of older people with dementia is expected to increase (Schneider and Guralnik 1990) and some proportion will continue to become board-and-care home residents, the stress of their care and their appropriateness to the small board-and-care home environment at advanced stages of the disease are important issues to address.

The data on residents in the Cleveland and Baltimore studies have revealed a population that is socially marginal to the dominant groups in society. They lack the characteristics and social ties that would place them within dominant groups and institutions. In many ways they fit the concept of surplus populations as described by Mizruchi (1987). As surplus populations, they have little influence in the society and may be perceived as burdensome. They are unable to effectively organize and advocate for themselves and do not fit neatly into the agendas of organized advocacy groups. This lack of advocacy makes them highly vulnerable to exploitation and abuse, the frequently cited reason that policymakers give to impose regulatory restrictions on board-and-care homes.

6 □ Social Supports and Relationships in the Homes

□ THE INTIMATE quality of social relationships is a consistently noted characteristic of small board-and-care homes (Dobkin 1989; Namazi et al. 1991; Sherman and Newman 1988). In the absence of regulatory oversight, small homes may choose clients on the basis of their type and degree of impairment, personal preferences, and compatibility with others in the home. Paired with the operators' positive orientation toward people, this flexibility may be critical to finding a good interpersonal mix. Limited oversight has allowed the social environment in small board-and-care homes to evolve in ways that might have been prohibited under strict rules and regulations (Appelbaum and Ritchie 1992; Segal and Hwang 1994). The relationships are not as bounded by institutionally structured roles and are therefore free to find their own definitions, ranging from familial to formal.

Newman (1989) attempted to identify the key structural and process components for assessing quality in private-pay (relatively expensive) compared with public-pay (funded largely or solely by residents' SSI payments) board-and-care homes. Process elements included maximum services and activities for residents and autonomy of residents in as many aspects of their lives as possible. To compare private and public homes on these elements, Newman interviewed and studied intensively five homes in New Jersey, New York, and Virginia, supplemented by short, on-site observations at twelve additional homes (Newman 1989). Based on this small and nonrandom sample of homes, Newman (1989) concluded that residents in private-pay homes were more likely than residents in public pay homes to receive enriching (e.g., recreation and social activities) and access (e.g., transportation, information, and referral) services that were responsive to their needs. Her findings were similar to those of other research that pointed to limited resources as a primary cause of poor quality (Dittmar et al. 1983). In spite of limited resources found among public-pay homes, she found no differences between public- and private-pay homes in the sensitivity and dedication of the staff (Newman 1989).

Reschovsky and Ruchlin (1993) used data from 205 board-and-care

homes serving the poor elderly in seven states to examine seven aspects of
board-and-care quality: resident oversight, fire safety, other safety, space
and privacy, supplemental services, resident and staff interaction, and
overall facility environment. Several of their findings have relevance for
the small homes discussed here. First, very small homes (four to six residents) outperformed larger homes with respect to resident and staff interaction. Overall, they found an inverse relationship between the size of the
home and the quality of social interaction. Lower staffing levels were also
positively associated with the quality of resident and staff interaction,
suggesting that the availability of staff may not enhance the quality of
interaction, but may have an opposite effect. They noted that some of the
dimensions of care important to the quality of life of residents (e.g., resident and staff interaction) bore no clear relationship to the cost of operating
the home and were inherently difficult to quantify.

The quality-of-life dimensions of social support and relationships are
the topic of this chapter. Various structural (formal and informal supports
and services) and process (home and familylike characteristics, activities,
interpersonal relationships) elements of board-and-care homes are examined, based on the interviews with operators and residents in Cleveland
and Baltimore. The analysis focuses on differences in these elements by the
size of the home, fee levels, race of the operator, and participation in
Project HOME in Baltimore. The longitudinal design and qualitative aspects of the study in Baltimore provide rich data on the social fabric of small
homes. These data are unique and differ significantly from most other
studies of board-and-care homes.

For board-and-care homes in the Cleveland study, information on formal and informal supports and social relationships was collected by asking
the residents who had helped them with activities of daily living (ADLs)
and instrumental activities of daily living (IADLs), coupled with a series of
direct questions about their relationships with the operator and with other
residents. In Baltimore, a profile of formal and informal supports was used
to determine all the individuals involved in providing care directly to the
residents or assisting the operator in their care. In addition to this network
profile, the operators were questioned about the homelike and familylike
characteristics of their facilities, activities, and interpersonal relationships
with residents.

Formal and Informal Support

The care of several adults with significant physical and/or mental impairments by a sole board-and-care home operator has been a source of concern (Newman 1989). Whether the operator, working seven days a week,

can meet all of the varied needs of the residents is a question closely linked to the quality of care in small homes. But do the operators of small board-and-care homes, such as those we studied, really carry the burden of care alone? Our research revealed that most operators have a network of support that provides a variety of services, either in the home or beyond its walls, in meeting the physical, social, emotional, and other needs of the residents.

A major feature of the first interview with the operators in Baltimore was a network profile of all the formal and informal supports involved in meeting the needs of residents in five categories: professionals coming into the home, resources and programs outside the home, paid nonprofessionals, kin and friends of the operator, and kin and friends of the residents. We will focus on two groups. The first includes professionals and formal programs that provide services to the residents, regardless of where those services are provided (i.e., formal, usually paid support). The second set of data reflects more-informal sources of support, such as the operator's family, residents' families, neighbors, and community groups. While operators reported a wide array of services (e.g., entertainment of clients, financial management, doing clients' nails), we focus on the most common services and those providing them.

From the five components of the network profile, we constructed an initial measure of the size of the total network described by the home operators as assisting them in any way in the care of their residents. The resulting index ranged from four homes having only one listed supporter to one home operator who listed twenty-eight. The median number of helpers listed in the network profile overall was nine. There were no statistically significant differences among various types of homes on this measure, with the operator of one of the smaller homes (three or fewer residents) claiming the largest network of twenty-eight helpers.

Formal Supports: Professionals, Programs, and Paid Services

A second measure, focusing on professionals and formal groups that assisted either by coming into the homes or helping clients outside the home, revealed smaller numbers of supporters. Two homes claimed no helpers from this group, and one home operator reported fifteen formal and professional supports. The median number of helpers in this category was four. There was a significant difference in the number of formal-sector helpers by the size of the home, with 37.5 percent of smaller homes having three or fewer formal sector helpers compared with 20.0 percent of the larger homes. None of the other comparisons showed significant differences.

Most operators reported several sources of formal support used by their residents, either within the homes or beyond their walls. Figure 21 shows that different groups tended to be mentioned within the home and outside, with three groups, social workers, nurses, and physicians, being mentioned in both cases. The percentages cannot be summed for the different bars for each type of support in figure 21, since some of those having help from these groups inside the home also had help outside. The total number of operators reportedly being helped by social workers was 74.8 percent; physicians, 45.6 percent; and nurses, 23.3 percent. Within the homes, social workers (including case managers) were by far the most commonly mentioned professionals, followed by physicians and nurses, who visited about one home in five. Other frequently mentioned groups included home health agencies, podiatrists, and "other professionals."

The formal supports provided within and outside of the homes were compared by the size of the home, the race of the operator, the average level of fees paid by the residents, and their participation in Project HOME. A number of significant differences emerged. Larger homes were more likely to have podiatrists making home visits. This is not surprising, since during a single visit to a larger home, a podiatrist could treat several residents. The frequency of physician visits to the homes varied by the race of the operator and by program participation. White operators and those not participating in Project Home were more likely to have physicians visit the clients in their home. This was expected, since those types of homes cared for an older and more frail clientele. Black-operated homes had greater participation in Project HOME and, as a consequence, were more likely to

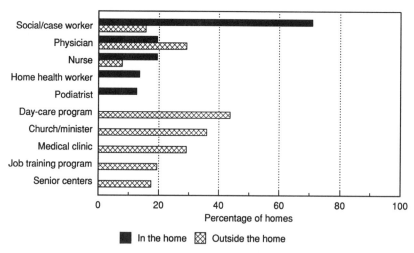

Fig. 21. Percentage of Baltimore Operators Receiving Formal Support Inside or Outside the Home

care for younger, physically healthier, deinstitutionalized people. Operators participating in Project HOME were also more likely to have clients using day-care programs. Again, this was not surprising, since participation in day-care programs is encouraged by the program.

Although not specifically listed in our network profile, ministers and church groups made visits to the homes. For example, an operator listed a church group as a formal support visiting her home. As a Mormon who used to take in young missionaries, she was still visited by these young people. She said, "I've been their Big Mama and they still come to me. My clients look forward to their visits and often ask when they will return." The operator felt that the visits and the interaction between the visitors and clients made an important contribution to the atmosphere in the home and to the comfort of her clients.

Not only did we inquire about the types of formal supports going into the homes, but also the frequency of their visits and the degree of helpfulness in the eyes of the operator. The ratings of their formal supports by the home operators in Baltimore ranged from "the greatest possible help" (3), to "makes no difference" (0) or "makes more work or gets in the way" (−3). Social workers, by far the most common type of visitor, also visited fairly frequently, with most of the operators reporting visits monthly or a few times a year. For example, one operator stated that the social worker did not come to her home unless there was a problem; she reported that this amounted to several visits per year. Physicians and nurses, on the other hand, were somewhat less frequent in their in-home contacts. While some operators reported daily visits by nurses, none did so for physicians. Physicians and nurses were equally likely to visit monthly or on a variable, as-needed basis. Home health agencies, however, were the most likely to make daily visits to the relatively small number of homes receiving their services. Podiatrists visited a few times a year or "as needed."

In terms of helpfulness, most operators rated their formal supporters in the home as being of the "greatest possible help." For example, one operator commented on the assistance provided by a nurse working with one of her clients. She was having difficulty in obtaining a pair of elastic panty hose (TEDS) for a client. The nurse willingly interceded for the operator with the pharmacy. The operator asked the nurse, "Why do they always give me such a hard time." The nurse responded, "I'm not sure, but everything is okay now." The same operator, during a later interview, said that she faced some difficulty in getting medication for a client. The pharmacy wouldn't accept the client's medical assistance card. The matter was finally resolved when a call was placed to the pharmacy by the patient's physician. Despite the generally positive view of operators and the pressures of social desirability, there was not uniform endorsement of the helpfulness of professionals. Operators rated a small, but noteworthy, minority of social/case workers and other groups as making "no difference" in their work load, and a few were rated negatively.

Difficulties often developed when operators learned that social workers had not been forthright in sharing information on the background and personal histories of clients they had placed. In several cases mentioned by operators, only after experiencing serious behavioral problems with a client did they discover a prior history of similar problems. For example, an operator refused to allow a former client to return to the home because he was not taking medications to control schizophrenia. She recounted her last encounter with him, "I asked him, are you taking your medicine? He told me, 'Don't need it, doctor said I don't need it anymore.' He came to use my phone to call his mother. They had some words. When I tried to talk to him about the phone call, he got angrier and then muttered something and then said, 'That's the problem with women!' I told him, 'Don't talk to me like that, you know that's no way to talk.'" Shortly after this encounter, the operator learned that the young man had killed his mother. The operator became very angry with the referring agency for not giving her information about the violence in the client's history. She said, "I gave them a piece of my mind. I want to know what their history is. I should know! I *need* to know! He tried to kill his mother three times. They knew that. They should have told me." In such cases, operators felt that they had been deceived by the referring professional and that their personal safety had been compromised by potentially violent clients.

Formal support outside the home included doctors and nurses, but the largest single support was adult day-care programs, reported by 43.7 percent of operators to be serving at least one of their residents (see fig. 21). Although we were anticipating traditional formal service providers in our questioning, the operators used a broader definition, listing church groups or ministers as the second most common group providing services to their residents outside the home (35.9 percent). This was followed by medical clinics, job training programs, and senior centers, all sites selected by significant minorities of the home operators in the Baltimore area.

The frequency with which the home operators used services outside their homes varied, based on the type of help received. Most used day-care or job training/rehabilitation programs daily or a few times a week. Senior centers were also typically used several times a week. Social workers outside the home were consulted anywhere from daily to a few times a year. Physician contacts outside the home were less frequent, a few times a year, while support provided by ministers or church groups ranged from weekly to monthly. Operators also used outside medical clinics monthly or a few times a year to meet the health care needs of residents. The frequency of the outside support, then, also depended on its type. A significant number of operators could be said to be receiving regular support through the day-care, job training/rehabilitation programs, and senior center services provided to their residents. These services are undoubtedly what enabled about one operator in four to hold outside employment while running a home. In fact, 73.0 percent of those who were employed outside the home also used such services.

As with helpers coming into the home, services consulted outside were rated highly favorably by the operators of the Baltimore-area board-and-care homes. One operator, affiliated with Project HOME, noted that the program was very helpful, stating that "training programs were very informative and well-directed at her needs." Another operator stated that she sees counselors to discuss problems and to get advice and uses whatever supports are available from Project HOME. This operator saw herself as responsible for bringing people together, clients with formal agencies and professionals, and clients with their families. She felt it was her responsibility to develop a support network and to see that it was maintained.

The fact that operators made distinctions between helpful and unhelpful supporters suggests that they were not simply responding in terms of social desirability and expectation. Although the great majority of operators perceived that their burden was lightened by the presence of a person or an institution making an effort at support, we cannot assume that this was always true.

An average helpfulness score for the total number of formal supporters named in figure 21 was calculated for each home. The scores on the resulting interval level scale (ranging from "the greatest possible help" (3) to "makes more work or gets in the way" (−3)) were then analyzed to see if there were differences between the homes based on their size, the fees charged to residents, the race of the operator, and their participation in Project HOME. The resulting scores were uniformly high, with nearly three-quarters (73.1 percent) of the homes giving their formal supports an average rating of two or more.

There were no significant differences in the operators' ratings of their formal supports based on the race of operator, the average fees, or their participation in Project HOME. However, operators of larger homes, on average, rated their more numerous formal supports as also being more helpful than did the operators of smaller homes. This is not surprising since, as noted in chapter 3, some of the larger homes we studied budgeted to pay for necessary expenses associated with larger operations (e.g., staff for personal care, cooking, and housekeeping).

Paraprofessional Support

Aside from these programs and professionals, operators reported on others who were paid to provide services, either inside or outside of the home. These paid nonprofessionals were present in over half of the homes

(52.4 percent), with a few operators mentioning as many as five or six such helpers. Larger homes had more persons in this category, including the staff persons described in chapter 2, but there were no differences by the level of fees paid by residents, the race of the operator, or the home's participation in Project HOME. Most commonly these paraprofessionals provided supervision to clients to enable respite for the operator (37.8 percent). Other paid services included housekeeping, yard work, and a variety of other tasks (see chap. 2). These were paid helpers (cooks, housekeepers, beautician/barbers, or backup caregivers) or friends and family of the operator who were compensated to perform these tasks. This group bridges the traditional distinction between formal and informal care. These paid nonprofessionals were apparently drawn from the informal network of the home operator rather than from agencies or community groups. Thus, for these board-and-care operators, there appears to be an intermediate category between what is traditionally thought of as the formal sector of care (paid professionals and nonprofessionals, agencies) and the informal sector (nonpaid family, friends, and neighbors).

Informal Support: Family, Friends, and Neighbors

The Operators' Family and Friends

The operators included some of what might typically be considered informal support in responding to our questions regarding services and professionals assisting their residents. We added questions regarding the operators' kin, neighbors, and friends and the family and friends of the residents to round out the profile of those who might be providing important support to the home's residents or the operators.

The great majority of the board-and-care home operators in Baltimore (90.3 percent) included at least one person from their families and friends as part of their support networks for running the homes. Most of the operators listed one to three family members or friends as supporting them in their work with residents, but a few mentioned as many as nine or ten. There were no statistically significant differences in the receipt of support from the operator's family and friends by the size of the home, the operator's race, the average level of fees paid by residents, or their participation in Project HOME.

The informal group most likely to be providing help to operators were their own children, often including those who were grown and living on their own. Nearly two out of three operators reported that at least one (and up to five) children provided them with some form of assistance (see table 14). Beyond the support from children, the operators' friends, spouses,

Table 14
Family and Friends as Supporters in Maryland Board-and-Care Homes

Relationship	Percentage Reporting Help	Modal Frequency	Helpfulness Rating (Mean)
Operators' kin/friends			
Child	64.1	As needed	2.86
Spouse	33.0	Daily	2.96
Sibling	18.4	As needed	2.78
Parent	11.7	As needed	2.66
Other kin	32.0	As needed	2.86
Friends	35.9	As needed	2.89
Residents' kin/friends			
Sibling	31.1	Monthly/few times per year	2.14
Child	21.4[a]	Weekly	1.95
Other kin	20.4	No mode	1.89
Spouse	2.9	No mode	1.33
Friends	8.7	Few times a year	2.07

[a]Difference by program participation (Project HOME participant vs. nonparticipant) is statistically significant ($p < .05$).

and other kin played a role in about one home in three. One operator referred to her home as a "family operation" because her sons, daughters-in-law, and grandchildren were all active in running the home and providing care to residents. An interviewer's field notes illustrate the cooperative nature of the home. "Trish, her daughter-in-law, seems to be the person on whom the operator relies a great deal and [she] has often been seen bustling about in the home, carrying laundry, tending to client needs, etc. Clients are always present. Physical therapy technicians and home health care nurses are in and out. All are greeted warmly and the feelings seem to be reciprocated. The operator refers to her husband as the 'fix-it man.' He assists with the personal care of the male clients at times, but apparently leaves client care to the rest of the family."

Although the percentage of spouses reported to be providing assistance (33.0 percent) was lower than the percentage of spouses reported to be living in the households (44.6 percent), the spouses differed from the other groups in that they were strongly concentrated in providing daily assistance to the operators. Apparently the spouses who provided assistance did so in a regular and significant way, gaining the highest rating on the helpfulness scale (averaging 2.96 on a scale ranging from -3 to $+3$). Both the siblings and the parents of the operators were also sometimes listed as helpers. These informal supports from the operators' personal networks appeared to be flexible in terms of availability, and they were highly appreciated. For all groups except spouses, the modal response was that help was provided on a variable, as-needed basis. That is, these groups constituted a network upon which the operator could call for a variety of tasks when the need arose. We do not know how often these helpers were actually called upon, but the operators rated the vast majority of them as of the greatest possible help (+3 on the helpfulness ratings) (see table 14). No differences were found in the operators' ratings of helpfulness based on the size of the home, the fees charged to residents, the race of the operator, or their participation in Project HOME.

Several of the operators spontaneously mentioned the existence of networks of operators that joined together to create informal support groups. One operator mentioned that the group to which she belonged met periodically to discuss problems in running a home. She said, "they [other operators] lay their cards right out on the table and then we discuss them." If members of the group felt "stressed out," they contacted each other and planned a "get-together." The meetings took place at one of their homes over coffee. She stated that these sessions had been very helpful to her in dealing with the stresses involved in providing board-and-care services.

Residents' Family and Friends

The social networks of the residents also played a role in providing support in the homes, albeit a lesser one. Over one-half (55.3 percent) of the Baltimore operators included at least one relative or friend of a resident in their support networks. Most mentioned only one or two such persons, and there were no significant differences by our usual comparison variables (i.e., homes of one to three residents compared with those with four to eight, homes operated by African American versus white operators, those with above and below average fees, and those that did and did not participate in the Project HOME program).

Siblings of residents were the most active group in providing some assistance, but fewer than one-third of operators reported the siblings of residents helping them or the residents in the past year (see table 14). They helped infrequently and were not viewed by operators as being as helpful as their own informal networks. The remaining supporters from the residents' networks were even less helpful, by operators' estimations. About one in five operators reported receiving help from a resident's child or other relative in the past year. While the children of residents tended to visit the board-and-care home somewhat more often than other kin, these visits ranged from several times a week, to yearly or less.

In comparing the involvement of the residents' kin and friends by the size of the home, the race of the operator, and the average fees, no significant differences were found. However, the children of residents were more likely to be involved in homes not participating in Project HOME. This reflects the lower probability of having children among Project HOME clients, with program participants more likely to be younger, never married, and deinstitutionalized from mental hospitals (see chap. 5).

Assistance from other resident kin also ranged widely in terms of its frequency, and both other kin and children showed a mixture of ratings on the helpfulness scale that pulled their average scores below 2.0. Relatively few residents had spouses or friends providing support. Those who did have them were assisted infrequently, and the few spouses of residents were rated by the operators as the least helpful of any group. Many of these findings regarding the low level of support from the residents' informal networks are best understood by the limitations of their personal and kinship networks, which were described in chapter 5.

Analysis of interviewers' field notes revealed both positive and negative experiences with the families of residents. For example, one operator discussed her frustration with family members and regulators, who always assumed that board-and-care home operators abused and neglected clients. She related an exchange in which a client's daughter, who placed her mother in her home, would "sneak into the home and look for incidents of abuse." She recounted that "one day I was caring for her mother, singing to her, when I turned and the woman was standing right behind me. It scared the daylights out of me. I told her to please knock in the future. She told me she wanted to be sure I wasn't hurting her mother. I told her this was my home and she would knock in the future." When the mother developed congestive heart failure, was hospitalized, and died, the daughter accused the operator of wrongdoing. "I was absolved of any wrongdoing, but this woman kept pressing the matter, telling everyone that she wanted to be sure others wouldn't be hurt the way her mother was."

Overall, operators gave high helpfulness ratings to their informal support network composed of their own and their residents' family and friends. Based on the average helpfulness rating scale described earlier, over four-fifths (83 percent) of the homes rated their informal supports as the greatest possible help (+3). While no differences were found when comparing homes by the race of the operator, the average fees, and their participation in Project HOME, operators of the larger homes were more likely to give higher average helpfulness ratings to their informal helpers.

In general, the ratings of help provided by professionals, service groups, and the operator's informal network suggest that they are fairly happy with most of the individuals and groups who provide support to them inside or beyond the walls of their board-and-care homes. This mixed support system provided a diverse set of services to benefit the operator, her residents, or both. This profile does not suggest an isolated caregiver, but rather a system, ranging from sparse to elaborate, to provide a variety of services, often in a flexible, as-needed fashion. Although this debunks the myth of the isolated caregiver, it should not be interpreted to indicate that the operator's needs were being adequately met (see chap. 4).

Residents' Reports of Help They Received

In Cleveland, select information on informal and formal supports was derived from the interviews with residents. Information on the informal supports came from questions about whether help was needed in performing the ADLs and the IADLs, whether they received help with these activities, and, if so, from whom. An individual's ability to perform basic self-care activities (such as feeding, toileting, and dressing) is reflected in ADLs (see chap. 5). Before suffering losses in ADL functioning, a disabled person faces more common problems in performing IADLs, tasks believed necessary to maintain an independent household (Kane and Kane 1990). These tasks generally require a combination of physical and cognitive ability. In Cleveland, the IADLs included cleaning one's bedroom, using public transportation, washing clothes, shopping, using the telephone, and managing money.

When residents needed help with ADLs (as shown in chap. 5, many residents did *not* need such assistance), they received it from facility staff, usually the operator herself. The "facility staff" also included members of the operator's family and paid staff persons. A major reason that persons were residing in the board-and-care homes was their need for assistance with IADLs. The relatives of the residents played a larger part in helping with these needs than with ADLs. Family members provided nearly three-quarters (73 percent) of the assistance required in the management of money (see chap. 3) and about half of the assistance needed with transportation and shopping. By contrast, operators provided the most assistance in setting up doctor's appointments (49 percent of the time by operators and 37 percent of the time by relatives). In cases where residents needed assistance with legal, physical health, or mental health problems, they received it through a combination of resources external to the homes (e.g., relatives, lawyers, senior centers, physicians, local hospitals, and community health centers).

In Cleveland, then, the residents reported that most of the help they received with ADLs came from the operator of the home, her family, and paid staff, supplemented by some assistance with IADLs from relatives. Formal providers of care were generally not involved in meeting these kinds of personal care needs but were mentioned by residents as being available when needed.

The operators of small board-and-care homes were not carrying the burden of caregiving alone. The operators and residents listed formal and informal supports both inside and outside of the homes. Overall, the operators in Baltimore viewed these supports as helpful, although cases of interference with the care they provided were reported for both formal and informal categories of supporters. The examples from interviewers' field notes illustrate various aspects of the social marginality experienced by the operators of small board-and-care homes. The next section focuses on the bonds that develop between the operators and residents, bonds that mirror neither traditional family or professional/client models.

Social Relationships and Social Interaction

Homelike and Familylike Characteristics

As was mentioned in chapter 1, a strong cultural preference exists in the United States for one's care to take place at home, to "age in place," and to "sleep in one's own bed" (Rubinstein 1995). This has contributed to the commonly accepted assumption among professionals, policymakers, and the public that homelike characteristics are desirable in nonfamily settings that house and care for dependent adults (see Aptekar 1965; McCoin 1983; Morrisey 1965; Skruch 1993). This preference is partially responsible for the growth of home and community-based services for dependent adults of all ages and its importance in long-term care policy.

Because it contains the word *home*, Johnson and Grant (1985) noted that the term *nursing home* connotes a small-scale, homelike setting for the care of those who can no longer care for themselves. A *home* connotes not only a place of residence but also a social unit formed by a family living together (Johnson and Grant 1985). Such units demonstrate primary group characteristics of small size, members living in close proximity and bound together by expressive functions, relatedness, and a long-term commitment. In addition, home and family are linked to the community, since many roles and activities are conducted outside the home (Johnson and Grant 1985).

Total institutions, on the other hand, are antithetical to the "home." As described by Goffman (1961), residents of total institutions experience a loss of privacy; little segregation between work, play, and sleep; and tightly scheduled routines and activities. Formal rules and a fixed schedule govern the daily activities of the residents and the staff alike. Moreover, total institutions serve populations that are intentionally segregated and isolated from the wider society, and the resident's stay is often a long one (Johnson and Grant 1985).

It is the stated goal of most nursing homes to provide a homelike setting for their residents. However, the setting is so strongly dominated by the medical model of care that it resembles a hospital rather than a home in most respects. Thus, few nursing homes have been successful in muting the institutional qualities of their environment (Johnson and Grant 1985). In reviewing the institutional qualities of nursing homes, Johnson and Grant (1985) stated, "Nursing stations are placed at intervals to maximize efficiency, and rooms are commonly arranged along corridors with adjacent doors opening off both sides. The space within rooms is not conducive to visiting by family and friends. Like hospitals, there may even be restriction on privileges. Since security is also a problem in large institutions, patients may be discouraged from bringing their personal belongings because of fear of theft, fire, and contamination. As a consequence, the impersonal aspects of a hospital may pervade institutions that are 'homes' for their residents" (Johnson and Grant 1985, 112).

Several studies have examined homelike characteristics in institutional settings for adults. Homelike environments have been linked to improved functional behavior (Knight et al. 1978; Carey and Thompson 1980), improved intellectual ability (Carey and Thompson 1980), and greater autonomy (Rotegard, Bruininks, and Hill 1981; Schultz 1987). Much of the literature on housing and residential care for dependent adults emphasizes the concepts of familylikeness and homelikeness and the advantages of such placements (Namazi et al. 1991; McCoin 1983; Morrisey 1965; Sherman and Newman 1988; Whorley 1978).

In this section we describe the ways in which small board-and-care homes are (and are not) perceived by their operators and residents to be homelike or familylike. Information on homelikeness and familylikeness comes from interviews with the operators and interviewer field notes in Baltimore and interviews with the residents in Cleveland.

In a previous analysis of the data from the Cleveland study, Namazi and his associates attempted to understand what constitutes "homelikeness" for elderly residents of small board-and-care homes. Their analysis built on nine conceptual dimensions of home identified in research conducted by Hayward (1975). Twenty-nine items from the interviews with residents were selected as representative of the variables in Hayward's nine conceptual clusters. They found that five factors contributed to the sense of homelikeness among the residents in small board-and-care homes: affinity, ambience, privacy and refuge, personalization, and operator's altruism. Four of the nine conceptual clusters were similar to those identified by Hayward (1975), while the altruism of operators was unique to the board-and-care environment.

The altruism of operators was felt by the residents and emerged as a theme in their discussions of homelikeness. When residents in Cleveland were asked why they felt their board-and-care home was like a family home, 18.3 percent mentioned the goodness of the operator as a primary reason. As was pointed out in chapter 4 and elsewhere (Eckert, Namazi, and Kahana 1987; Sherman and Newman 1988; Skruch 1993), the altruistic motivation for helping others is a recurring theme among board-and-care home operators.

The residents in Cleveland were also asked several direct questions about homelikeness and familylikeness. Over two-thirds (68.8 percent) of the residents answered that their board-and-care home was like a "home" rather than "just a place to live." When asked if their residence was "like a real home," 35.8 percent answered that it was somewhat like a real home, and over one-half (50.9 percent) answered that it was very much like a real home. In referring to other people living in the home, over two-thirds of the residents (67.9 percent) answered that they were "just like family." There were no significant differences in the responses to these questions on the basis of the size of the home, the race of the operator, or the average fees paid by the residents. Thus, from the perspective of the residents interviewed in Cleveland, homelikeness and family-likeness were dominant features of their living environments.

In the third interview in Baltimore, operators were asked about their perceptions of the atmosphere in their own homes. In response to two open-ended questions, operators listed the ways in which their homes were like a family, followed by the ways in which they resembled a nursing home. They were then asked to indicate where they thought their home fit along a nine-point scale, ranging from "home" (1) to "nursing home" (9). Their responses ranged from 1 to 6, with a mean of 1.98 and standard deviation of 1.41.

There were no significant differences between operators in how they rated their homes on the home-nursing home continuum on the basis of the size of the home, the race of the operator, or participation in Project HOME. There was a difference, however, based on the fees charged to residents. In homes charging higher fees, the operators rated the environment as more like a nursing home. This difference may reflect a tendency, noted in chapter 3, for higher-fee homes to act more "medical" by keeping records on the residents' medications and medical conditions. In spite of this difference, the operators of small board-and-care homes generally thought of their homes as familylike.

To open-ended questions, operators volunteered a number of characteristics that made their homes either like a family or like a nursing home (table 15). A maximum of three responses were coded for each. The most frequently mentioned characteristics that made board-and-care homes like families in the eyes of the operators included sharing activities (56.7 per-

Table 15

Operator Characterizations of What Makes Home
Like a Family or Like a Nursing Home

Characteristic	Percentage of Operators Mentioning ($N = 103$)
Like a family	
Sharing activities	56.7
Showing love and affection	35.6
Quality caring	33.3
Bonds like own kin	18.9
Residents use whole home	14.6
Treating residents as individuals	13.3
Residents have autonomy	12.2
No schedule	7.8
Shared tasks	7.8
Fight like a family	4.4
Pets	1.1
Like a nursing home	
Assisting with medications	51.1
Providing close supervision	20.0
Monitoring medical problems	16.7
Arranging services	5.6
Paperwork	2.2
Foley catheters	2.2
Ethnic diversity	1.1
Keeping residents busy	1.1

cent), showing love and affection (35.6 percent), the high quality of caring (33.3 percent), and bonds like those with their own kin (18.9 percent). Other less frequently mentioned characteristics included residents being able to use the whole home (14.6 percent), the operators treating their residents as individuals (13.3 percent), supporting the autonomy of the residents (12.2 percent), having no fixed schedule (7.8 percent), the sharing of tasks (7.8 percent), and, to a lesser degree, fighting like a family (4.4 percent), and having pets in the home (1.1 percent).

When operators were asked what made their homes like nursing homes, they focused on medically oriented services. Assisting their residents with medications (51.1 percent), providing close supervision of the residents (20 percent), and monitoring the residents' medical problems (16.7 percent) were the most frequently mentioned activities that made their homes like a nursing home. Other activities mentioned by the operators included arranging services for the residents (5.6 percent), doing paperwork (2.2 percent), maintaining Foley catheters (2.2 percent), ethnic diversity in their homes (1.1 percent), and keeping their residents busy (1.1 percent) (see table 15).

The interviewers' field notes provided additional insight into how operators viewed the home–nursing home continuum. When one operator was asked to place her home on the continuum, she placed it in block number three, nearer to the family end of the continuum. She stated that she offered better and more individualized care than did a nursing home. She based this assessment on an experience with a client who had come to her home to stay until the family was able to place her in a nursing home. After the client was moved to a nursing home, the operator often visited her to see how she was getting along. She was upset, however, by the lack of care the client was receiving. Noting that the client was blind, the operator stated that she was often left to bathe herself or to figure out what was on her meal tray. One of the resident's relatives made a big sign and placed it over her bed, notifying nursing home personnel that the client was blind and needed help. The operator concluded that there was really no comparison between nursing home care and the personalized care she offered.

In another instance, an operator became offended when the interviewer referred to her home as a "board-and-care home" and then asked if any characteristics of her home were "like a nursing home." The operator stopped the interviewer to comment, "I don't think of my home as a board-and-care home. We are just one big family!" Similarly, when asked if there were aspects of her home that resembled a nursing home, she said that her home was a "family, we do things together, sit together, eat together, talk together." When conflicts developed in the home, the operator and residents held a "family reunion." At these special meetings, residents and the operators discussed grievances, such as one resident feeling that the operator was giving too much attention to another. In discussing the function of these meetings, the operator stated, "Family reunions are good for us, they bring us close together." Not surprisingly, this operator placed her home at the family end of the continuum (block number one), even though she recognized aspects of care similar to those in a nursing home (supervision of residents and helping them with their medications).

Even for those operators who provided medically related services, the familial style of delivering care pervaded their comments. One operator, who routinely used medical terminology when discussing clients (e.g., referring to clients as patients and talking about departures of residents as discharges), also identified her home in block number one of the continuum. Even though she monitored blood pressure, treated decubiti, gave Foley care, and performed other medically related services, she saw the one-on-one care she provided as akin to what a family would do. In this regard, she stated, "This is a home. We are with them, pushing them through, not just giving treatment." In another instance, an operator stated that there was no way she could compare her home with a nursing home, since her home was "a family." Even though some of her clients were very dependent on her for care, similar to that provided in a nursing home (e.g., an elderly bed-bound client on oxygen), she believed that she was more "individualized" in her approach to care. She also noted that her children were very attached to the clients and interacted with them on a regular basis. She became particularly attached to clients without family, stating, "I tend to take them under my wing." In such cases, her close attachments resulted in keeping severely impaired clients longer than she could have anticipated. She stated that she often wondered at what point to say "no more." She laughed, however, and added, "I haven't reached that point yet, though."

Both the operators and the residents of these facilities perceive them to be homelike and familylike. Within small board-and-care homes, the members are living in close proximity and are bound together by expressive functions, relatedness, and commitment that denote home and family. Variations in the size of the home, the race of the operator, the average fees charged to the residents, and their participation in Project HOME in Baltimore had little impact on these dominant themes. The next section details the types of relationships and social interactions that give meaning to the notions of home and family in the board-and-care setting.

Social Interactions

Several types of relationships exist in small board-and-care homes. The primary interactions between the operator and each resident have been described by some authors as the most important (Sherman and Newman 1988; Namazi et al. 1989). There are relationships among the residents themselves and interactions between the residents and others who are in the homes on a regular basis (e.g., the operator's family and friends, formal and informal supports, and in some cases, paid staff). The residents' social networks of family and friends, although they may be limited in comparison to those of other populations (see chap. 5), are also worthy of attention. In addition, there are relationships between the residents of small board-and-care homes and the neighborhoods and the larger communities in which they are located.

Feelings and Attachments

Reports by the residents in Cleveland and the operators in Baltimore indicate their feelings about the other people living in the home. Residents in Cleveland were asked a number of questions concerning their perceptions of relationships in the board-and-care homes, with responses displayed in table 16. When asked about the degree of closeness among the people who lived in the home, 38.5 percent said that they were very close, and another 40.4 percent felt that people in the home were somewhat close. There were significant differences in the degree of closeness on the basis of the size of the home (48.5 percent of residents in the smaller homes felt a great deal of closeness compared with only 29.6 percent of the residents in homes of four to eight) and on the race of the operator (in homes operated by an African American, 25.5 percent of residents reported feeling some closeness, compared with 44.9 percent in the other homes). Over three-quarters (77.1 percent) said that others living there were usually comfortable to be with, and 17.4 percent said that this comfort was felt only sometimes. The board-and-care residents mentioned friendliness, shared backgrounds, kindness, helpfulness, trust, and dependability as reasons for their sense of comfort with others living in the homes.

Table 16
Residents' Feelings about Relationships
in the Cleveland Homes

Response	Percentage Responding ($N = 218$)
People who live here feel closeness[a,b]	
A great deal	38.5
Some	40.4
Not much	11.5
People who live here are just like family	67.9
People here are comfortable to be with	
Usually	77.1
Sometimes	17.4
People help one another	77.5
People have fun together	61.9
People understand your worries	
Usually	45.4
Occasionally	25.2
Not at all	23.9
There is someone here you can trust	90.4
Do you feel like a stranger here?[a]	
Never	75.7
Sometimes	18.8

[a]Difference by home size (1–3 vs. 4–8 residents) is statistically significant ($p < .05$).
[b]Difference by race of home operator is statistically significant ($p < .05$).

According to the residents in Cleveland, the people in the home helped one another somewhat or a great deal (77.5 percent), had fun together (61.9 percent), and understood the residents' worries (usually, 45.4 percent; occasionally, 25.2 percent). There was almost always someone in the home in whom the residents could trust (90.4 percent). When asked whether they ever felt like a stranger in the home, 75.7 percent of the residents said that they never felt that way, but 18.8 percent had felt that way at some time. Significantly more (82.5 percent) of the residents in the smaller homes said that they never felt like a stranger, compared with 69.6 percent in the larger homes.

From the Baltimore study, an interviewer's field notes indicated the strength of the attachments between residents and operators. One resident had lived in the board-and-care home since 1966 and was considered a member of the family. When the resident's lawyer asked him how he wanted to settle his estate, he chose to leave it to the operator, rather than to his sisters. In another instance, the resident was aware that he had become more of a burden to the operator after returning from a hospital stay. The operator told him that she expected to give him more care, and that in time he would be better. The client said to her, "You know missy, I had to come home. You love me here, you love me here."

In the Baltimore homes, the operators responded to a number of queries about their attachments to residents (see table 17). Almost all of them (96.6 percent) reported having felt close to residents in the past year, and most (85.4 percent) claimed to have felt close to nearly all of their residents in that time. For some of the operators these attachments created problems. Some (39.5 percent) said that they had kept a resident for too long a time (i.e., beyond the point where they needed more [or less] care) because of their feelings for them. Others (33.7 percent) had faced a problem getting over the death of one or more residents to whom they were attached. Supporting the altruistic motivations of some of the operators (see chap. 4), 54.7 percent reported that they had kept someone who couldn't pay all or part of their normal fees for services, and nearly three-quarters (71.8 percent) claimed that they would keep current residents, even if they were unable to pay in the future, because of emotional bonds with their residents.

There were no significant differences between operators on these responses when compared by the size of the home, their race, the fees they charged, or their affiliation with Project HOME in any of their responses to these questions, with the exception that Project HOME operators were significantly less likely to have experienced problems getting over the deaths of residents. It may be that residents who were participating in Project HOME were less likely to die, since they were younger and less

Table 17
Operators' Attachments to Residents in the Baltimore Homes

Response	Percentage Responding ($N = 90$)
Felt close to residents in past year	96.6
Have felt close to nearly all residents	85.4
Being close to residents has caused problems	34.4
Kept someone too long because of feelings	39.5
Kept someone who couldn't pay all or some of fee	54.7
Would keep current residents if unable to pay	71.8
Had problem getting over death of resident	33.7[a]

[a]Difference by program participation (Project HOME, non–Project HOME) is statistically significant ($p < .05$).

physically impaired (see chap. 5). The operators reported the deaths of significantly fewer residents (33.3 percent versus 66.7 percent) in homes that were participating in Project HOME. However, some of the difference is probably due to the operators being less likely to become attached to the residents who exhibited disruptive behaviors related to mental illness. What is most striking about these findings is that the nature and character of interpersonal relationships seems to be uniform across homes, regardless of distinctions based on the size of the home, the race of the operator, the amount charged for services, or their affiliation with Project HOME.

One of the operators in Baltimore told the interviewer that hugging and touching were an important reason why she grew closer to some residents than to others. When asked if these feelings of closeness caused a problem for her (e.g., keeping a client longer than she should), the operator responded, "I prefer them to be with me. They need me. I will care for them till the end." In another case, the client in question was a drug and alcohol abuser and had left the home "without even saying goodbye." The operator said that she felt sad that the resident left despite these difficulties, adding, "Separating really hurts."

Another operator became teary when she discussed a "very lovable" client she had cared for in the past. The client had moved from Florida to the board-and-care home to be near her niece and nephew in Baltimore, since they were the only relatives she had. She developed congestive heart failure and was hospitalized. The hospital called the operator and told her the resident would not eat. The operator hired an aide to stay with her other clients while she went to the hospital three times a day to feed her client. "The little stinker ate every time without any problem. Then, she would grab my hand and say, 'You're not going to leave me now, are you?'

The last time I saw her, she told me, 'Stay with me tonight, I'm not going to see you tomorrow.' I just couldn't stay. She died that night."

Residents' Family and Friends

Board-and-care home residents generally had fewer kin than do others in the population, although most of them did have some family members (see chap. 5). The data from both studies provide information about visiting among the residents and their families and friends, giving us some insight into these relationships.

The residents in the Cleveland study were asked a series of questions about visits with family members. As presented in figure 22, nearly three-quarters of them (72.5 percent) reported receiving visits from relatives. There were significant differences in the percentages of residents visited by their relatives when they were compared on the basis of the race of the operator (60.8 percent in homes operated by blacks vs. 76.0 percent), and on the fees paid, with fewer visits by relatives in lower-fee homes (66.4 percent) than in higher-fee homes (78.4 percent). More than one-third of the residents (36.8 percent) reported visitors at least once a week, and 21.2 percent reported having visits from family members less often but at least once a month. Nearly one-quarter of the residents (22.9 percent) did not feel that their relatives visited often enough, and a few (1.4 percent) said that they visited too often! Nearly half of the residents (45.0 percent) said that they sometimes went out of the home to visit their relatives.

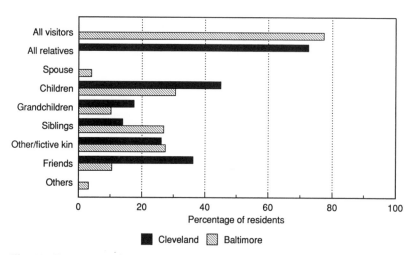

Fig. 22. Percentage of Board-and-Care Home Residents Having Various Types of Visitors

The most common visitors to the Cleveland residents were their children (45.0 percent reported receiving this type of visitor). The residents were more likely to be visited by their children in white-operated homes (51.5 percent vs. 23.5 percent) and in the higher-fee homes (58.5 percent vs. 30.8 percent). Some of these residents received visits from their grandchildren (17.4 percent), their siblings (13.8 percent), and other relatives (26.1 percent). More of the residents in the smaller homes (34.0 percent) said that they received visits from other relatives than did residents in larger facilities (19.1 percent).

In addition to having ongoing relationships with family members, most (65.6 percent) of the residents in Cleveland said they had friends outside the board-and-care home. Of these, more than one-third (36.2 percent) said that their friends visited them in the homes (see fig. 22), and 8.7 percent felt that friends did not visit them often enough. About one-fourth of the residents (23.9 percent) left the homes to visit their friends.

We asked the operators in Baltimore about the people who visited the residents in their homes. For nearly one-quarter of the residents (22.7 percent), the operators did not report any visitors. One-third of the residents (33.0 percent) had only one regular visitor. The most frequently reported interval for these visits was weekly, followed by a few times a year. When residents received visits, most of them were made by family members or quasi- or fictive kin, although friends (10.5 percent of residents had this type of visitor), church members (2.3 percent), and volunteers (0.9 percent) also called on them.

Children of the residents in Baltimore were also their most common visitors (30.6 percent of the residents had children visit). There were significant differences in the children's visits when residents were compared by the race of the operator (22.6 percent in homes with black operators vs. 45.8 percent), by the fees paid (22.9 percent in low-fee homes vs. 38.9 percent), and by the home's participation in Project HOME (37.7 percent in homes not participating vs. 16.1 percent). Overall, 10.2 percent of the residents received visits from grandchildren. The proportion of these visits differed by the size of the home (7.8 percent in smaller homes vs. 18.7 percent) and by the race of the operator (17.8 percent in homes with white operators and 6.2 percent in those with black operators). Only 4.1 percent of the residents were visited by a spouse, but over one-quarter of them (26.9 percent) received visits from their siblings. None of these figures are surprising, given that some residents had fewer kin than did others their age (see chap. 5). Over one-quarter (27.4 percent) of the residents received visits by people who we describe as quasi- or fictive kin. They were not any of the relatives discussed above, nor were they reported as friends. Although we do not know much about the quality of the interactions among the residents and their visitors, most of them do not appear to be estranged from family and friends.

One Baltimore operator told the interviewer about her efforts to reunite one of her clients with her family. Apparently the family was afraid the resident's cancer was contagious. The operator was able to satisfy their concerns enough so that she began taking the resident to visit the family regularly. On these visits, she took bags of groceries, since the family had very little money. The operator said, "[Y]ou know how cheap chicken is and greens. It's not much, just the little extra we may have around here, or if there is a sale. Those kids go crazy when they see us now."

On the other hand, some relationships between residents and their families were not good. An operator described an interaction between a resident who had Alzheimer's disease and her daughter. She said that she had never witnessed such cussing between daughter and mother, but said the client was domineering and "just plain mean." The daughter apparently reached her breaking point and pushed the mother, who pushed back. The operator tried to intervene but only made things worse. The client called the police, who assumed the operator was abusing the resident. They left when they discovered that it was the client and her daughter who were fighting. The operator was upset about having been presumed to be abusive and having the neighbors aware of the confrontation.

Interactions in the Community

Sherman and Newman (1988) found that an important element in the familylikeness of the small adult foster care homes that they studied was interaction of the residents with the neighborhood and the larger community. In Baltimore, the operators were asked about the involvement of the residents in their communities. Over three-quarters (75.5 percent) of them said that their residents had some contact with neighbors or others in their communities. The most frequently cited reasons for the lack of community involvement of the residents were impairment (62.5 percent) or that they were busy (20.8 percent). Most of the contacts the residents had in the community occurred daily or several times a week.

To further detail this issue, we asked the operators about the types of contact that residents had with people in the community, with the opportunity to provide up to three responses. The types of contacts the operators described included visiting with the neighbors outside, over the phone, or in their homes, mentioned by 79.1 percent of those answering. The residents also participated in shared activities with other people in the community (14.3 percent), and in some of the homes, neighbors brought gifts or treats for them (4.4 percent). Residents in 2.2 percent of the homes ran errands for their neighbors.

According to an interviewer's field notes, one operator said that neighbors on her side of the street knew that she took care of people. The neighbors were often her eyes, watching the clients when they were out in the community and reporting to her when something was not quite right. Another operator told the interviewer that he taught his clients how to apply makeup, so that they would make a better impression when they interacted with others in the community.

Activities

Some authors have suggested that many board-and-care home residents spend their days just sitting around doing nothing, which is assumed to be detrimental to their well-being (Dittmar et al. 1983; Dobkin 1989; Newman 1989). The data from the Cleveland and Baltimore studies offer glimpses of day-to-day activities in these small homes.

Passing the Time

In Cleveland, the residents were asked several questions about what they did with their time. While 10.1 percent of them said that they never went out and another 6.9 percent went out very infrequently, 61.9 percent went out of the home at least once a week. It is likely that many of the residents who did not leave the home were unable to do so because of physical or cognitive impairments. The activities that the residents pursued when they went out included going for walks, eating and drinking, visiting others, and going to church, health appointments, shopping, and senior centers or clubs. Few of the residents owned cars. Therefore, when they left the home, they walked, used public transportation, or relied on the operator, family members, or friends to transport them. Many of them (44.0 percent) said that they would like to get out more often, and it was most often poor health or lack of transportation that prevented them from doing so.

Interviewers also asked the residents in Cleveland how much time they spent watching television and how much time they spent sitting around the home, not doing anything. In response to the first question, nearly one-tenth (9.2 percent) of the residents said that they did not watch television at all, more than half (56.4 percent) watched from one to four hours a day, and about one-third (32.5 percent) spent five to twelve hours in front of the television. Watching television involves some stimulation, whatever its value, but in response to the second question, more than one-quarter (26.2 percent) of the Cleveland board-and-care home residents said that they spent eight or more hours a day sitting around doing nothing, supporting the perceptions of some authors (Dittmar et al. 1983; Newman

1989). Another one-quarter (22.0 percent) said that they never sat around but instead found ways to fill their time.

When the residents were asked what they did in their spare time, some said that they watched television, reflecting responses reported above, but they also did other things. Some of the residents had hobbies, including sewing and other handwork and cutting coupons. Others wrote letters, read, talked to friends and other residents, or went for walks. Residents reported that they liked to listen to the radio, and a few said that they participated in sports, including basketball and bowling. Some of the activities reported by the residents were helpful to others, including baby-sitting and doing chores in the home.

Doing Chores and Helping Others

Doing chores in the home may help people feel useful and connected to the group (Streib, Folts, and Hiler 1984). This orientation toward participation is different from the total dependency fostered by nursing homes. Some of the Cleveland residents (40.4 percent) said that they helped with chores. Washing dishes and helping to keep the house clean and neat were the most frequently reported chores. Of those residents who said they did chores, one-half (50.0 percent) wanted to do them, and another 28.5 percent did chores for their own benefit (i.e., to stay in shape, to keep busy). The remaining 20.5 percent of these residents said that they were asked to do chores, were required to do them, or they needed money.

In Baltimore, the operators were asked what things their clients did to help them in the board-and-care homes. Some of the clients (13.5 percent) did nothing to help the operators. More than one-half (56.3 percent) of the operators reported that the residents helped them by doing household chores. Yard work was the next most frequently mentioned task (12.7 percent), followed by making snacks (5.6 percent), running errands (4.0 percent), helping with child care (2.4 percent) and other, unspecified tasks (5.6 percent). We did not ask the operators whether they required the residents to help them, so that the amount of choice the residents had in doing these chores cannot be determined.

An operator in Baltimore described one of his residents as extremely helpful and considerate. The client allowed the operator to sleep late on Saturdays by taking care of his four-year-old son. She also did the dishes, helped to prepare meals, and did other chores in the home.

These caregivers were also asked about the things their residents did to help each other. Nearly one-third (31.0 percent) of the responses involved residents doing errands or getting things for each other. While 11.5 percent of the residents checked on each other or got help for each other if it was needed, 8.8 percent helped each other with their clothing, and 13.3 percent did other tasks for their peers in the homes. Another 35.4 percent of the responses given by the operators were that the residents did nothing to help each other or that this question was not applicable, most likely because the residents were not able to assist each other because of physical or mental impairments or because it was a single resident home.

Shared Activities

In their studies of foster care homes for adults, Sherman and Newman (1988) found that the operators interacted more with their residents than the residents interacted among themselves. An interviewer's field notes from the Baltimore study reveal the pivotal nature of an operator's role in her board-and-care home. "While this operator is a very pleasant, loving person, I have come to realize that she has plenty of what she refers to as 'horse sense.' It has been my impression that the home revolves around this woman. Clients seek her out when they are not sure others are going to take care of their needs to their satisfaction. Family members seem to have a great deal of respect for 'Mom.' When minor or major emergencies occur, she is the one to coordinate and reassure."

In the Baltimore study, the operators were asked about activities shared among the members of the board-and-care households. Activities were shared more frequently between the operator, her family members, and the residents than they were among residents, supporting the findings of Sherman and Newman (1988). Some residents were not able to participate in activities with each other, because they were too frail or too cognitively impaired to do so.

Figure 23 shows the percentage of homes sharing the list of activities, as reported by the Baltimore operators. Eating together (operators, their family members, and the residents) is a shared activity that was mentioned by 84.4 percent of the operators. This activity was more common in homes operated by African Americans (91.7 percent vs. 67.9 percent for white operators). A similar question asked of operators in Cleveland revealed that 70.5 percent of them ate with their residents, and all of the homes with multiple residents reported that the residents ate together. Fewer operators (62.2 percent) in Baltimore said that their residents ate meals together frequently, while 21.1 percent of them said that the residents were unable to do so.

The operators in Baltimore were also asked about exchanging cards and gifts with residents. Most of them (84.4 percent) said that they did so, but only 26.6 percent of the operators claimed that their residents exchanged gifts or cards with each other. In nearly one-fifth (18.9 percent) of these homes the residents never exchanged gifts or cards with each other, and 44.4 percent of the operators judged that the residents were unable to

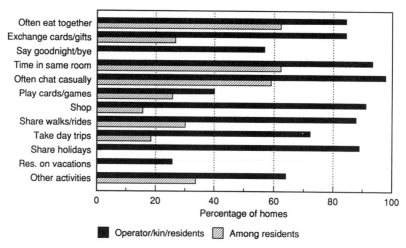

Fig. 23. Activities Shared by Operators, Their Families, and Residents in the Baltimore Homes

participate in this activity because of poverty or frailty. For some of these marginalized residents, the lack of emotional bonds with each other limited this type of interaction.

As figure 23 shows, saying goodnight or goodbye to each other is another ritual that takes place in more than one-half (56.7 percent) of the board-and-care homes. One of the Baltimore operators told an interviewer that when she started to kiss one of her residents goodnight, the resident said, "I don't go for any of that kissing stuff." The operator did not try to kiss her the next evening, and on the third night the client asked, "Where's my goodnight kiss?"

In response to another question in this series, most of the operators (93.3 percent) reported that they spent time in the same room with the residents, while the clients in fewer (62.2 percent) of the homes spent time together in the same room (see chap. 2). Again, a significant minority of the residents (21.1 percent) were unable to do so.

We also asked the operators if they and their family members chatted casually with the residents and played cards or games with them. As was true for other shared activities, the operators were more likely to participate in these activities with their residents than the residents were likely to do together. Almost all (97.8 percent) of the operators reported frequently chatting with residents, while 58.9 percent of them said that the residents chatted with each other (24.4 percent were unable to do so). As figure 23 also shows, residents in larger homes were more likely to have conversations with each other (92.8 percent vs. 52.7 percent), perhaps because there were more opportunities to do so. An operator described how she was able to facilitate interactions between residents. One client, who was confined to her room most of the time, was taken to the family living area a few times a week for short periods of time. In the interim, the operator would include the resident in as much activity as possible by sending other residents in to visit or by arranging visits from outsiders.

Nearly one-half (47.7 percent) of the operators said that they never played cards or games with their residents, with black operators significantly more likely to say this (50.0 percent vs. 42.9 percent of white operators). Only about one-fourth of the operators (25.6 percent) said their residents participated in these activities together, and the same proportion were not able to do so.

Another series of questions concerned activities shared by the board-and-care home residents and the operators outside the homes. Nearly all (91.1 percent) of the operators said that they and their family members shopped with their residents, with those in the homes participating in Project HOME more likely to do so (97.5 percent vs. 86.0 percent), perhaps because their residents were less physically frail. In only 15.6 percent of the board-and-care homes in Baltimore did the residents go shopping together.

A high proportion (87.8 percent) of the operators said that they went for walks or rides with their residents, with this activity more likely to take place in homes operated by African Americans (91.7 percent vs. 78.6 percent in homes with white operators). Only 30 percent of the residents participated in walks and rides together, with significantly more of them doing so in larger homes (64.3 percent vs. 23.6 percent) and in the homes that were participating in Project HOME (37.5 percent vs. 24.0 percent). The same pattern holds true for other activities (see fig. 23). While 72.2 percent of the operators said they took day trips with their residents, it is not surprising that only 18.4 percent of the residents took day trips together, given their lack of resources.

Many of the operators and their families (88.9 percent) shared holidays with the residents, and perhaps surprising to those who think of the board-and-care homes as businesses, one-fourth (25.6 percent) of the operators took residents on vacations with them. According to an interviewer's field notes, one client told her caregiver that she was afraid of being forgotten during the holidays. The operator described how she and her family "took Christmas" to the resident, who had recently entered a nursing home. Another operator told an interviewer that she believed that one of her residents was "holding together for his ninety-sixth birthday." Ten of his family members were expected to be there to celebrate with him in the board-and-care home, including some from Florida.

Nearly two-thirds (64.0 percent) of the operators reported that they shared other activities with their residents, while one-third (33.7 percent) of them said that residents shared other activities together. The other activities the operators listed included trips to the mall, concerts, plays, and sporting events, eating in restaurants, singing, and doing projects together, such as crafts and gardening. One operator in Baltimore told the interviewer that her son often took the male clients fishing or involved them in similar activities.

The interviewers' field notes provided glimpses of life in small board-and-care homes through their own eyes. One interview took place in the kitchen of a board-and-care home in Baltimore with two residents present. The interviewer arrived as the operator and the residents were watching their favorite soap opera, and the interview could not begin until the show was over. The interviewer described the interactions among the home's occupants as good, marked by relaxed and jovial conversations. She noted a genuine affection between these three members of the household. The operator's young grandson came in to visit during the interview. The clients were excited and happy to see him, fussing over him as if he were their own grandson. The child ran to them before he went to his grandmother. On another visit to a home an interviewer found the residents sitting out in the yard, talking among themselves. The operator told her that this usually happened every day that the weather was nice. The residents would congregate and socialize after returning from day-care.

Loneliness and Boredom

Authors who reported that board-and-care home residents just sit around and do nothing were concerned that they were lonely and bored (Dittmar et al. 1983; Dobkin 1989; Newman 1989). In the Baltimore study, the operators were asked what they did to help alleviate loneliness and boredom for their residents. In response to a question, "Is loneliness a problem for your clients?," more than one-half (51.1 percent) of the operators said that loneliness was *not* a problem for any of their residents, 24.4 percent said it was problematic for some or for a few, and 14.6 percent of them said that it was a problem for most of their clients. There was no variation in their responses on the basis of the size of the home, the race of the operator, the fees for service, or participation in Project HOME.

The operators were asked to list up to three things they did to help their residents avoid feeling lonely. The most frequent response was spending time or socializing with the residents (58.9 percent). Forty percent of the responses involved developing activities for residents; providing games, puzzles, magazines, and newspapers; promoting interactions with pets; facilitating religious activity; and involving residents in all aspects of life in the home. Another 40 percent of the responses concerned activities outside the home, including going to senior centers, to day-care, and to church; taking day trips; and going for rides in the car. Some of the operators (24.4 percent) said they used music or television to help alleviate loneliness in clients, and other activities included having outsiders come to visit (8.9 percent), providing special treats for residents (5.6 percent), involving clients in doing chores in the home (4.4 percent), and reminiscing with residents (3.3 percent). A few of the responses to this question (4.4 percent) were that the residents were very busy, and therefore, presumably, they didn't have time to be lonely.

A similar set of questions concerned boredom experienced by the residents. These questions elicited similar responses from the operators, and there was no variation based on our usual comparison variables. They judged that boredom was a problem for none (58.9 percent), some (18.9 percent), or most (10.0 percent) of their residents. A little more than one-tenth (12.2 percent) of the operators said they did not know if boredom was a problem for their residents.

Providing music or television (35.6 percent) and taking clients out to senior centers, to day-care, to church, on day trips, or for rides in the car (35.6 percent) were the most frequently mentioned activities provided by the operators for relief from boredom. Thirty percent said that they spent time with residents to keep them from being bored; 22.2 percent provided games, puzzles, magazines, and newspapers for this purpose; and 13.3 percent developed activities for the residents. Approximately one-tenth (8.9 percent) of the operators said they brought outsiders into the home to keep clients from being bored, and the same proportion provided special treats for the residents. The only significant difference between homes was on this variable when comparing homes by fees for service, with higher-fee homes providing more special treats. Otherwise, paying more for care did not make a difference in the activities the operators arranged to alleviate boredom in their residents. A few of the operators (4.4 percent) said that they had residents do chores to alleviate boredom, and 10 percent of them said that the residents can do what they want, implying that they are free to be bored or they can find things to do on their own. One operator told the interviewer that she felt her residents were too busy to be bored or lonely. She said, "Home is where they come to relax." They usually ate dinner together, then went to their own rooms for the evening.

An interviewer described how she was taken into the kitchen of the board-and-care home, where she found a client eating the breakfast she had prepared for herself. The small kitchen, where all of the members of the household spent a lot of time, was apparently the hub of activity in the home. In addition to a television, the tables and counters in the room were filled with items (puzzles, games, toys, and a gumball machine) to "keep their minds working," according to the operator. The operator had what she referred to as her "ugly wall," filled with drawings by her grand-children and her clients, notes, calendars, and crafts done by the residents.

□ THE SOCIAL context of the care provided in the small board-and-care homes is critical to the quality of life for residents and operators alike. Both the supports received by these groups and the nature of their bonds with one another can enhance or detract from the care given.

The operators of small board-and-care homes were not isolated care-givers; they had networks of both formal and informal supports to sustain them. The formal supports included professionals, programs, and others who provided assistance within and outside of the home. The informal supports included the families, friends, and neighbors of the operators and, to a lesser extent, the families and friends of the residents. Overall, the operators viewed their formal and informal supports as helpful. The families and friends of residents were rated by the operators as much less helpful than the other groups, more often interfering or creating more work for the operators.

These support networks represented a mixed support system that pro-vided a diverse set of services, benefiting the operator and her residents on an as-needed and flexible basis. This is not to say that all of the operators needs were being met (see chap. 4). Many operators expressed dissatisfac-tions with service availability, financial resources, and health care coverage for their clients. In terms of the concerns voiced in the literature (Dittmar et al. 1983; Newman 1989), however, it appeared that most operators did not provide care in isolation, devoid of support from formal and informal sources.

For the operators and residents of these small board-and-care homes, definitions of quality go far beyond the easily quantifiable dimensions of the physical environment, staffing, and services. The familial and home-like characteristics of the environments were the core themes defining quality of life and quality of care. The operators and residents alike viewed the homes as family homes, unlike nursing homes in almost every respect.

The operators played a pivotal role in coordinating the system of formal and informal supports and in creating the familylike atmosphere in the home. The altruism of operators and the quality of caring in their relation-ships with their residents was surprisingly uniform across the homes, regardless of their size, the race of the operator, the average fees paid by the residents, and their participation in Project HOME in Baltimore.

Although the residents of the homes had fewer kin than others in the general population, most had family members and friends with whom they maintained contact. Residents also had contacts with neighbors and others in their communities. While some were without such contacts, because of their mental and physical impairments or the lack of family and friends, these were not totally isolated and estranged people.

The residents of small board-and-care homes were involved in a range of activities both inside and outside the home. While residents engage in activities among themselves, activities were shared more frequently with the operator and her family members. For some, this was expected, since they may be the only resident in the home or too frail or cognitively impaired to interact with other residents. Activities typical of a family home, such as eating together, exchanging gifts, and spending leisure time together were common among the operator and residents. Although operators reported that loneliness and boredom were experienced by some residents, they did not appear as problems of immense proportion.

A final vignette from an interviewer's field notes in the Baltimore study demonstrates the strength of the feelings and attachments that can take place among the people who live in small board-and-care homes. The operator described the recent death of a former resident living in a nursing home. She said, "[T]he nurses told me it was quick, she just closed her eyes." The operator became misty-eyed as she recalled the details of the funeral she arranged for the resident. She and her family (her mother, her children, and an aunt) made donations for the headstone. The cemetery donated the plot, and the operator's minister performed the service. The operator bought the resident "a pretty pink dress, she wore the ring I gave her . . . she looked good." She said that the resident was always afraid she would be buried in 'potter's field.' "I told her that would never happen, and I was true to my word."

7 □ The Future of Small Board-and-Care Homes

□ SMALL BOARD-AND-CARE homes stand in the uncharted territory between family and institution, public and private organization, and independent living and medical dependency. In addition to describing this environment in greater detail than has been possible in the past, the studies in Cleveland and Baltimore have delineated many of the possibilities and problems arising from the marginalized status that is faced by the operators, the residents, and those organizations responsible for funding and regulating smaller board-and-care homes.

Our findings also relate to the futures of other settings in the long-term care continuum that share this marginal ground between home and institution. Concerns about cost containment, quality of care, and providing community-based alternatives appear as part of the contemporary debates on child care, homelessness, and welfare reform. Society is grappling with alternative approaches to protect and nurture dependent populations of all ages and types. Decisions in these areas highlight schisms in our ideologies regarding the degree of help the less fortunate deserve, societal responsibility for those in need, and the balance of individual autonomy against oversight in providing care.

In this chapter we outline key findings, summarize the evidence on marginality, and discuss the core issues in the possible, alternative futures for the small board-and-care home industry. Homes, such as those we studied, face a turning point in the next few years, and the decisions that are now being made regarding their regulation and funding will dramatically shape their future. These decisions are part of the tug-of-war among various stakeholders in the reform of health care (Dougherty 1992).

Summary of Major Findings

Our goal in conducting this research centered on gaining insights into the realities of the internal environment of (i.e., the insider's perspective on) small board-and-care homes. Our research was not representative of all that is called board-and-care (or given myriad, related names), because of the designed limitations of our research methodology. Moreover, variation across states in the regulatory and financing climate faced by operators of these small homes means that drawing a comprehensive picture of the board-and-care industry would be nearly impossible (Dobkin 1989; Hawes et al. 1993; Reschovsky and Ruchlin 1993). We do draw some conclusions regarding the small, "mom-and-pop" homes that contrast, often sharply, with the public image of such facilities. These small homes represent a center of concern for policymakers in many states, who are deciding how best to accomplish their regulatory goals (Applebaum and Ritchie 1992; Dobkin 1989; Newman 1989; Segal and Hwang 1994). What are the realities of the small board-and-care homes that we studied?

Topical Findings

The physical environments of most of the homes were similar to family environments that care for dependent persons. Houses had seldom undergone major modifications; children, pets, relatives, and the residents intermingled in the living spaces; rules were informally made and enforced, often to protect the privacy and safety of residents; and a variety of services, akin to those promoted for assisted-living facilities, were available in most homes on an "as needed" basis. Our interviewers rated the physical environments of most homes as good to excellent, in contrast to the negative images presented in the media.

The single bedrooms found for most of the residents differed from a typology developed by Newman (1989). She described smaller homes (typically run by one person) as requiring double occupancy of bedrooms, sharing of bathrooms, little privacy, and few activities and services for residents. In the homes we studied, although the bathrooms were shared, as they are in family homes, services and activities were generally available. Although we did not measure the size of these single bedrooms, interviewers' descriptions of them did not portray cramped or squalid quarters.

The economic situation in many homes was tenuous, with operators receiving little money above what they reported as their expenses. This excess, when it existed, constituted the profit or payment to the home operators, who lacked a regular salary in most cases, as well as any employment-related benefits. The loss of one resident through death or relocation often meant that an operator had no profit margin or had to dip into personal resources to make ends meet. Many operators complained of the extra, unreimbursed expenses associated with the care of their residents, such as damage to furniture and linens from incontinence or inadequate funds to purchase clothing or over-the-counter medications.

Despite this tenuous position, most of the residents in these small board-and-care homes paid small to moderate monthly fees in comparison to those of other care alternatives. These low fees often took all of the money the residents had to support themselves (less a specified amount for personal spending, in many cases). Operators in this largely unregulated market faced difficult decisions regarding whether to take a needy resident with limited funds that might give them a small profit or to turn the resident away and hold the bed for a more lucrative resident. Many of the poorest residents would have been unable to purchase services, let alone room and board, for their modest monthly stipends from SSI without the board-and-care system.

Operators disavowed money as the central motivation for their work, preferring to emphasize the service component of caregiving. This altruism is a general orientation toward life, as indicated by the comments of one operator. She said, "One person can't move the world, but that person can make a difference. The neighbors bring things to my clients, because they know they appreciate it. I know this lady who called her grandkids 'bitches and bastards,' but those kids know not everyone thinks of them that way. They know me and they know that I care!" Because of their altruism, the board-and-care system absorbs a large number of dependent adults who would otherwise be homeless or cost society much more money for their care in institutional settings, such as mental hospitals, prisons, or nursing homes.

The operators of the homes in Baltimore were surprisingly unburdened by the demanding work they had undertaken, perhaps because they were a self-selected group. Although many did report problems in their work, those problems were varied, and none were characteristic of most of the operators who responded to our interviews. Nearly three-quarters of the operators in board-and-care homes had previously worked in formal health care settings, and many claimed that they could better serve residents' needs at home, without the bureaucratic demands of the larger organization. The current operators were confident of their ability to provide good care, and most drew lines delimiting the types of clients they were unable or unwilling to accept into their homes.

The corps of operators in both cities was mature and aging. This raises concerns about whether the future will bring sufficient motivated operators into the small board-and-care industry for it to remain a viable component of the care system for dependent adults. Changing roles and opportunities for women and the professionalization of caregiving in some sectors are pressures against the replacement of the current provider group (Harmon 1982; Sokoloff 1992). Our research did not permit us to answer the question of whether the grass-roots board-and-care industry will pass from the scene with the retirement of the current cohort of operators.

We were somewhat surprised at the willingness of busy operators in both locations to spend the time required to participate in the study, which involved four interviews and numerous telephone calls in Baltimore. Some of the Baltimore operators were sad when data collection was ending, having become attached to the interviewers who were sincerely interested in their lives and work. One remarked that she felt her participation had some psychological benefit for her, because she could talk about her situation without fear of being judged. Unaware of others involved in board-and-care work, she said, "I don't know who the people are nor where they are, but knowing that there are others out there like me makes me feel less alone."

Residents in small board-and-care homes were often multiply impaired, with both physical and mental or cognitive limitations. In the Baltimore study, mental illness was especially prevalent because of the placement efforts of the Project HOME program. Problematic residents seem to circulate among board-and-care homes. Many of them came from other homes, and many who left quickly, probably because of behavioral problems, moved to another, similar home. This process seems to continue until a particular resident finds an operator and a home environment that can manage the troublesome behavior.

Many of the other residents we studied had moderate to long stays in homes, where they appeared satisfied with their situations and well integrated into the household. Resident satisfaction must be weighed, however, against their likely options, which may have included homelessness, institutionalization, or living with distant or unwelcoming relatives. For most of these individuals, independent living in their own house or apartment in the community was not a viable alternative. Given this context, resident satisfaction with board-and-care homes, an option that most people would find basically undesirable, is more understandable.

Social interaction patterns in the homes revealed the central role of the operators, who served as a hub of interaction. The operators do not work in isolation, as it might initially appear, but have flexible networks of social supports, drawn from both formal and informal sources, to provide specific skills and supplement their time and energy. Most of the small homes in our studies could be described as homelike, with sharing of space and routine activities, much as occurs in family residences. In addition, these interaction patterns and homelike characteristics were consistent across various types and sizes of homes we examined.

Attachment between operator and resident can be a double-edged sword. The familylike interactions between the operators and their clients in the homes are thought by many to encourage attentive and personalized care. We heard many stories of operators making extra efforts to provide foods, activities, or situations to meet particular residents' needs. Yet the attachment also prompts operators to sometimes overlook their own needs and limitations. Some operators had obviously kept residents who were quite impaired and probably would have been removed for nursing home or psychiatric hospital care by social workers. For example, after suffering a heart attack brought about by the demands of caregiving, one operator was again ready to accept clients. She claimed that she was now going to make an effort to care for her own needs, instead of only worrying about others.

Diversity

Despite selecting a relatively narrow band of homes from the overall board-and-care spectrum for study (i.e., those housing eight or fewer residents and having a coresiding home operator), we detected significant diversity among the homes in Cleveland and Baltimore. This diversity in how the homes operated bespeaks their origins as a grass-roots development. The absence of regulatory oversight has meant that the homes have distinct flavors and textures not generally found where rules and regulations foster the type of institutional sameness seen in nursing homes. We purposefully examined certain aspects of diversity, expecting to find differences among the homes.

Home Size

The selection of smaller homes, those that often remain outside the current requirements of state licensure, was purposeful, since less is known about these homes than the larger, more institutional end of the board-and-care spectrum. Our focus on size appears to have been justified, because we found differences in homes and their operators even between the smallest (three or fewer resident) homes we studied and those that housed only up to eight residents. In homes with more than eight beds, we anticipate that the fundamental nature of the environment and care would change toward an institutional model very rapidly.

Larger homes in most of the prior research have shown elements of institutionalization not present in the homes in our sample (Reschovsky and Ruchlin 1993; Segal and Hwang 1994). Descriptions of staffing, for example, were not suitable for most of our homes, where the caregiving work is done by the operator and her kin, with the occasional assistance of respite providers, neighbors, and professionals. Seldom do the small homes have workers in them who might be labeled as staff in the usual institutional sense.

Our contention that small homes are different appeared to be substantiated not only by comparison to research conducted by others but also by several findings of these studies. Homes with four to eight residents were more likely to have paid staff working in them, the residents were more likely to have double rooms, and the homes were more likely to run on fixed schedules. Residents in these larger homes paid higher fees, and family members more often paid privately for the care. The operators were also more likely to keep written records, reflecting a more institutional orientation.

Operator's Race

Since the family caregiving literature had suggested important differences in how African Americans cared for their own elders (Belgrave, Wykle and Choi 1993; Deimling and Smerglia 1992; Taylor and Chatters 1986), we anticipated that homes with white and African American operators might differ in some important ways. It is noteworthy that more African Americans undertook work as board-and-care providers than would be expected from their percentage in the population.

There were some significant differences in the homes and their operation. First, homes operated by whites were more likely to include the operator's spouse and a household pet. Children were also more common, but the difference in this variable by race was not statistically significant. African Americans who ran board-and-care homes were more likely to share living space and bathrooms with their residents and, perhaps because of this, were somewhat more likely to have rules about privacy and behavior in the home. African American operators also received lower ratings in some areas of quality of the physical environment, as might be expected given their lower socioeconomic status.

More important differences appeared in the area of economics, where, not surprisingly, homes operated by white providers received more income and had higher profits. In part, this difference is a result of the larger average size of the homes operated by whites, but it also reflects differences in the fees charged. Whites were also more likely to have served older and frailer women, perhaps warranting higher fees for more intensive, personal care. Differences in fees and profits between African American and white operators in Baltimore would have been higher in the absence of Project HOME, which provided substantial subsidies, pushing many homes operated by African American participants into the higher-fee category. African American operators were less likely to keep records of everyday expenses and report worries about finances, perhaps reflecting some difference in their approach to money. African American operators almost universally reported motivations of service, rather than monetary gain, in selecting their work. They were also more likely to mention interpersonal aspects of their work as key to good performance, including liking people and the capacity to provide tender, loving care.

Perhaps the differences were, overall, less than might have been expected. For example, there were few differences in social interaction and interpersonal aspects of the home's operation according to whether the operator was white or African American. Many of the distinctions we did discover may have related more to the difference in the size of the homes, participation in Project HOME, or socioeconomic factors (i.e., fee levels) than reflect ethnic differences in orientations to caregiving.

Level of Fees Paid by Residents

The amount being paid for board-and-care services is almost always related to whether the funds are public or private. The level of fees has also been connected to select aspects of quality (Lyon 1993; Newman 1989). Certainly the fees paid could be expected to make some difference in facilities and services offered and in the profits available to the operator once services have been provided.

Operators in lower-fee homes in our Baltimore study did show some differences. They were slightly (but not significantly) less likely to have modified their homes and slightly more likely to find some problems with their homes currently. Only two services were less often available in lower-fee homes. The remaining aspects of the physical environment, including the quality ratings by interviewers, did not differ significantly by the fees being paid by residents.

The operators of higher-fee homes were younger, had more education, more often worked outside the home, and had been offering services for fewer years than their lower-fee counterparts. This paints a picture of a potentially emerging group of operators who may move the board-and-care industry toward professionalization and profit motivation. Nonetheless, none of the examined attitudes demonstrated substantial differences by the levels of fees being charged, arguing against this conclusion.

Residents in higher-fee homes were, in general, older, more physically frail, and more likely to be female. In Baltimore the picture was confounded by the fact that subsidies for residents participating in Project HOME placed those homes in the higher-fee bracket. Despite these distinctions in the residents, however, there were almost no differences in the patterns of interaction and support in homes charging lower or higher fees.

In general, the fees paid by residents for their housing, meals, and care were modest by comparison with those for nursing homes or even assisted living (Kane, Wilson, and Clemmer 1993). The range of fees paid in both cities was, however, quite broad, including the "elite" homes in Baltimore, charging their residents $1,500 per month or more. The fee levels in our "elite homes" approach the charges for nursing home care, but operators are largely using the funds for amenities and services, rather than paying staff for medical care. The presence of these elite homes reinforces the economic diversity among small homes and emphasizes the fact that not all board-and-care homes consist of marginally poor operators caring for poor and marginalized elders. It is notable that these elite homes, having the option to pick and choose their clientele, cared only for white and elderly residents. The elite homes are probably the ideal of many regulators in terms of physical plant, services, and amenities. The dilemma is that only those who can afford this care out-of-pocket are able to avail themselves of this option.

Participation in Project HOME

The Baltimore homes that participated in this integrated program received subsidies, case management services, and operator training. The homes, because of the program's history, were more likely to house younger, mentally ill residents and include more residents and operators who were African American. Regulators more frequently visited operators with residents in Project HOME, because they had scheduled case-management responsibilities.

Comments to the interviewers indicated that the reactions to Project HOME were mixed. Some operators did not like the time required to attend meetings, but others found the support from the program helpful. As one operator participating in the program told our interviewer, she had provided a home to many people over the years, but only within the last five years had she been paid for the service. A friend had told her about the Project HOME program. Her discussion of the program was *very* positive, stating that the training programs were informative and well directed at meeting her needs. She also expressed a desire to open another home but stated that it was very difficult to gain access to "start-up funds."

There were also some areas in which expected differences did *not* appear. Attitudes of the participating and nonparticipating operators were quite similar, as were the physical environments of the homes. The residents in participating homes were more similar than expected in terms of functional impairment. In both sets of residents, physical and mental limitations were linked with social marginality, placing them in a highly vulnerable position.

Other Aspects of Diversity

The dimensions we used to examine diversity among the homes in our studies are, themselves, interrelated. These interrelationships sometimes form noteworthy patterns that explain differences, or lack of differences, in the findings. For example, participation in Project HOME was more common among African Americans, who also operated smaller homes (as mandated by Project HOME). White operators, who tended to run somewhat larger homes, charged higher fees and were more likely to house elderly clientele. Thus, distinctions by the operator's race, size of the home, the level of fees being charged, or participation in Project HOME are not mutually distinct. Had multivariate analyses been conducted, we anticipate that many of the significant relationships would have disappeared, with their covariance explained by indirect effects. Caution should be exercised, therefore, in interpreting the results, since it is not clear which of these (or other) interrelated factors might be the "cause" of differences between groups.

One implicit goal in this analysis was to draw contrasts between the environments of small board-and-care homes in Cleveland and in Baltimore. The two states differed in terms of their economies and regulatory structures at the time of the studies, leading to expectations that there would be some noteworthy differences between them. Our findings overwhelmingly support a conclusion that they were more similar than different. In some instances comparisons were made difficult by lack of comparability in the data collected. In most of the areas in which comparisons could validly be drawn, responses were remarkably similar.

Operators, for example, reported similar problems occurring in their homes and comparable levels of fees being paid for services. Avenues for entry into board-and-care work and motivations for continuing in it were strikingly parallel for the two operator samples. The demographic profile of the operators in the two cities was, with the exception of race, remarkably similar in terms of education, marital status, age, and health care employment experience. The profile of the residents in the two cities was also quite similar and mirrored findings in other states (Hawes et al. 1993).

Similarity

Despite the diversity in the homes that we studied, there were significant areas in which there seemed to be minimal difference among them. These themes tie the smaller homes together into a rather distinct phenomenon, differentiating them from the larger homes studied by other researchers.

Services

Across locations, home size, operator race, the level of fees, and participation in Project HOME (in Baltimore), there was remarkable similarity in the set of services that were available to the residents of the homes. The services reached beyond rooms and meals to include varying levels of personal care, transportation, and supervision. The service package appeared to be fairly comprehensive in most homes, with not all residents availing themselves of all possible services (e.g., financial management or transportation).

In our discussions with operators, they seemed to assume that undertaking the care of a resident involved providing whatever mix of services would be needed to maintain that person in safety and comfort. The fact that neither smaller homes nor those receiving lower fees had fewer services speaks to the interpersonal intimacy involved for coresident operators in small homes.

Operator Attitudes

Another area that was striking for its consistency was the attitudes of operators. Comparisons on attitudinal items about the burden of caregiving, the importance of money, and motivations for working in board-and-care showed few distinctions. The operators overwhelmingly rejected the view that what they were doing was running a business, preferring instead to focus on the service aspect of their work. As one stated, "If I hit the Jackpot, I would buy another home to care for old people."

Often the underpinnings of these motivations were strong religious beliefs, but we did not ask structured questions about religiosity. As one operator stated, she felt it was her duty to care for residents since, "The Lord had it to be this way." A strong desire to help others in need, apparently unsatisfied by work in institutional caregiving environments such as hospitals and nursing homes, prompted operators to take residents, some of whom could pay only minimal amounts for their care or required intensive supervision.

The homes are operated on the basis of altruism rather than for financial gain, in most cases. Like other care providers in the irregular economy, operators of small board-and-care homes negotiate "a tenuous balance between love and money" (Enarson 1990, 239) in their work with residents. Disdain for money, relative to the rewards of service, points up a critical issue for the future work force in paraprofessional caregiving. If work contexts do not permit individuals to gain a sense of satisfaction from providing care of good quality, it may turn highly motivated persons away from this type of work. The inability to provide good quality care because of the demanding work load has been pointed to as a key to work dissatisfaction among nursing home aides (Bowers and Becker 1992; Diamond 1990). Permitting sufficient workplace autonomy to allow expression of these motivations may improve quality of care and address problems of worker motivation in direct care to dependent adults in a variety of settings (Tellis-Nayak 1988; Vesperi 1983).

Homelike and Familial Characteristics

Based in a physical environment that encouraged such an orientation, relationships within the small board-and-care homes could be described as familylike. Residents were encouraged to personalize their rooms and to use common areas to the extent their physical status permitted. Operators shared activities with their residents, usually including them in family-style meals and in birthday and holiday celebrations. Activities in common living areas included conversation, television watching, and craft and game activities, much as would occur in a household comprised of kin. This represents the more normalized milieu that has been advocated for dependent persons (Morrissey 1982; Sherman and Newman 1988).

The key role of the operator in this quasi-familial system was reinforced by our research. Just as others have shown (Sherman and Newman 1988), residents felt closer to the operator than to one another, and the operator served as the hub of the home's social network for residents and family members alike. This social responsibility adds to the pressure on operators already pressed to deal with personal care and supervision of residents, as well as the cooking and cleaning for a multiperson household.

Often unexpected linkages were forged between operators and residents. An African American operator in Baltimore took in an Italian lady, aged eighty-one. Despite concerns at first because of the race difference, the operator said, "I asked her to look beyond my color and just see if I am good to her." Now the client has become family to her. "When my brother comes to visit, the first thing he asks when he walks in that door is 'Where is S.?' " When the resident became paralyzed from a stroke, the operator visited her daily in the hospital to conduct range-of-motion exercises. Once discharged, the operator shared a bedroom with her, to meet her physical needs during rehabilitation.

Possible Futures: Issues for the Board-and-Care Industry

Caring for the Needs of Marginal, Dependent Adults

As a society, we can anticipate an increase in the number of dependent adults needing care to manage their everyday lives. This population requires assistance in everyday activities, not medical treatment; maintenance in the least-restrictive environment, not warehousing in large institutions; in other words, care rather than cure. The conditions creating their dependencies are generally chronic and long-term, with some being degenerative over time. Thus, the management of their lives is a long-term-care concern, unlike an acute illness to be medically treated.

Families continue to do the bulk of caring for dependent adults through private networks (Soldo 1981; Stone, Cafferata, and Sangl 1987). The problem rests with those lacking the kin support necessary to meet their needs, a potentially growing percentage of the dependent adult population (Treas 1977). The residents in small board-and-care homes are striking in their lack of close kin, those who would be most likely to provide the intensive care they require.

Philosophically, society has moved away from large institutions for the mentally ill, in favor of smaller, less medical community sites. Such community settings better match a quality of life to which society aspires for all of its members. The "normalized" environment in a small home, such as a board-and-care home, is assumed to break down barriers between these "differently abled" groups and the general population and promote new living skills or the maintenance of existing ones (see Blake 1987; Donahue and Oriol 1981).

The changes of the deinstitutionalization movement were initiated prior to the current budgetary pressures affecting the federal government and most states. Now lower cost remains a key consideration for any care alternatives that might be proposed (CSSP 1988; Doty 1993). The deinstitutionalization movement intended for communities to absorb their own dependent adults, either back into family systems or into smaller, community-based treatment and support programs. These programs never materialized in many communities (Donahue and Oriol 1981; Morrissey 1982; House 1989). Instead, the mentally ill were left to fend for themselves, with many finding refuge in board-and-care homes (Blake 1987; Dobkin 1989). Now similar efforts may be underway to deinstitutionalize the elderly to respond both to public preferences and to public cost considerations (Doty 1993).

The term *underclass* emerged in the 1960s to describe a highly marginalized population that is urban, of low income and social status, and physically, socially, and psychologically isolated (Baca Zinn 1989). Current debates on welfare reform, education, and health care indicate that society has not come to terms with either the reasons that such marginal populations exist (e.g., are they at fault or is their status the result of social factors over which they have no control?), or what the society should do about them. Many of the board-and-care home residents described here as socially marginal fit into the underclass of American society.

Questioning the entitlement to socially funded benefits for those not seriously in need as a means of trying to control costs may erode the already tenuous base of public support for programs financing custodial care, such as board-and-care homes. The residents are not the most impaired in the population, but they lack critical social supports that often bridge the gap between independence and dependence. Given their marginal social backgrounds, this group of underclass individuals, lacking education, close and supportive kin, pensions, and even Social Security retirement benefits in many cases, are the most vulnerable to falling through the safety nets for health and income as they are currently constituted.

Assuring Quality in Board-and-Care Homes

Newman (1989) raised the question of whether homes can provide both homelike settings and high-quality care. Other research (Dittmar et al. 1983) has questioned whether quality can be maintained in public-pay homes, in which operators are receiving only minimal fees to care for dependent adults.

It is important to counteract the notion that all unregulated or public-pay homes are of poor quality. Our research suggests that there are good-quality small homes available in the board-and-care field, including public-pay homes receiving low fees. Our samples may have been skewed toward the higher-quality homes because of the refusal by operators in ramshackle houses or with questionable caregiving skills to be interviewed because of fear of discovery by the authorities. We uncovered many homes in which members of our research team felt they could have lived quite comfortably, had their health and personal circumstances required such care. The interviewers told us that their views on the homes had been transformed during the course of four visits. During early interviews, they noted clutter, noise, or the faint odor of urine in some homes. By their fourth visits, however, these aspects of the homes had paled in comparison with the vivid pictures of attentive, personal care and affection between operators and their residents.

The essential goal of quality is to assure optimal outcomes for the clients of the board-and-care homes. Yet given the difficulty in determining what constitutes a desired outcome for the population currently housed there, researchers, like regulators, generally fall back on aspects of the structure (e.g., staffing, buildings that meet safety needs) and process (e.g., resident activities, community involvement, and autonomy) features of the home as the basis for assessing quality (Newman 1989; Reschovsky and Ruchlin 1993; Segal and Hwang 1994). Unfortunately, this approach overlooks the very dimensions of care and interpersonal relationships that are most important to the quality of life of the residents. It is our failed capacity to measure what is central to quality of care in board-and-care homes that pushes us toward regulating and overseeing quantifiable aspects of the structure and staffing.

Dougherty (1992) suggests six key values at stake in debates about reform of health care, but which relate well to custodial care of dependent populations. These values are respect for the dignity of persons; caring in therapeutic relationships; protection of the least well-off; service to the common good; containment of costs; and simplicity in the system of health care provision. Our findings suggest that many of the small board-and-care homes already meet these goals, with others having the potential to do so if additional support was made available to them.

We asked our interviewers, during a debriefing session, to describe the characteristics of the best homes they had visited. None of them had difficulty in identifying a number of homes that stood out from the others, and their comments focused on the behaviors and attitudes of the operators. Among their descriptions of what made these homes special was

> They offer a comfortable, family atmosphere where the clients can come in and be themselves. They can argue, they can care for each other and move about the house with autonomy. The operators respect the individuality of the clients. These operators recognize that some of these clients just don't want to [be involved in day care or the community], and they respect that and support them and give them their space and accommodate to the needs of the client.
>
> Most of the houses were clean. They weren't necessarily dust free or organized efficiently all of the time. There might be clutter in places, but it was livable. It was a place to sit and relax and enjoy. [There was a] family environment in these homes. The clients were involved in all aspects of the home. They ate together, they talked together, they shared things together. These operators really have the clients' best interests in mind. They consider their preferences. They involve them in meal preparation. All of [the best] operators were able to build and preserve self esteem.

Another emphasized autonomy, stating that

> [T]he best homes, the ones I would want to live in, are where the operators control their clients the least. [Clients could say] I would rather watch TV or read a book, [rather than] go to a senior center. There may be some guidance, because the clients have Alzheimer's disease or schizophrenia, but [daily life] is not controlled. [The operators] are open hearted, and they really care about their people and protect them and defend them from the system. This is personalized care. People really care about them. They are not bodies.

A third noted that for an excellent operator she interviewed,

[T]here was just no limit to what she will do for her clients. Be it recreation, things that she thinks will help them enhance their lives, or make them better physically. There is just nothing she won't do.

When the interviewers were asked by one of their peers if they thought that the frailer residents, who were *not* housed in the "best" homes, were better off than they would have been in nursing homes, the unanimous response was "Absolutely."

The evaluation of quality is clouded by the various perspectives of policymakers and program administrators, social service personnel, the public, the media, and those living within the homes. The outsiders tend to view the issue in terms of risk and cost, trying to minimize both, while those inside tend to focus on the interpersonal dimensions, dealing only with finances as a necessary evil. Attempts to weed out poor-quality operators and homes by imposing measurable standards for quality may miss the key issues for everyday life of insiders by focusing on structural elements, such as doorway width and sprinklers.

Our evaluation of the quality of board-and-care homes (i.e., the facilities and the operators) are somewhat subjective and far from comprehensive. Serious questions remain regarding how best to assess quality (Newman 1989; Reschovsky and Ruchlin 1993). According to the parameters we evaluated, however, the quality of care appeared to be high and, in answer to Newman's question, was provided in a homelike setting.

Several authors (Dittmar et al. 1983; Newman 1989) have claimed that the number of services would be restricted in lower-fee homes, presumably on the assumption that fewer staff persons could be hired to attend to the needs of residents. Our results in very small homes, however, show only two less-essential services (i.e., protection from outsiders, barber and beautician services) were more common in homes in which the residents paid higher fees (see chap. 3). When a single operator manages the care of a small number of residents, the number of services appear to be unrelated to the fees that they pay.

Certainly our society would prefer to see all of its dependent populations housed and cared for in comfortable and safe circumstances. There remains, nonetheless, the harsh reality of growing resistance to paying more taxes to support social programs for dependent adults, especially the most marginalized groups, such as the mentally ill. When we compared the physical environments of the homes we studied to a middle-class, suburban standard of living, many of them were found wanting. That seemed to be the strategy of the U.S. House Select Committee on Aging in its exposé treatment of board-and-care homes (1989). If, on the other hand, we used the alternatives available to the populations housed in board-and-care, such as their prior housing in poorer parts of the city, life in mental hospitals, or residence with unwelcoming friends or family, the environment they experienced in all but the worst board-and-care homes seemed acceptable or good.

The quality of care in these homes is treated differently than quality of caregiving within family groups. The fee-for-service basis of the relationship seems to automatically remove assessment of quality from the standards that would be employed for families caring for frail elders at home. It remains apparent that utilization of standards of quality devised for some other type of setting, such as nursing homes, will find many small board-and-care homes deficient. And, as will be apparent, the issues of quality, regulation, and financing are difficult to disentangle.

Regulating Board-and-Care Homes: The Issue of Risk

On an organizational basis, our society has dealt piecemeal with the financing and regulation of facilities to care for the dependent populations in its midst. One set of agencies and programs have developed for the elderly, another for the developmentally disabled, yet another for the physically disabled under age sixty-five, and so on. These agencies and programs have had varying levels of success in generating funding and public support for their agendas, resulting in wide differences in support to the various populations. For example, a fairly sophisticated system of agencies and supportive group-living settings have emerged for the developmentally disabled. These settings, often housing small numbers of disabled adults, are staffed by trained professionals and are linked to a network of sheltered workshops and services (Taylor and Racino 1991).

The mentally ill poor have fared much worse, often ending up living on the streets or, if they are lucky, in board-and-care homes. The poor and marginalized elderly have also fared poorly under this system. Fears regarding the potential cost of lowering the safety net to catch these dependent adults has precluded more than spotty coverage of their needs (Doty 1993).

In spite of unanswered questions, many states are now engaged in hot debates regarding the licensure, certification, or other forms of regulation for smaller board-and-care homes (Dobkin 1989; Stone and Newcomer 1986). The first unanswered question is whether regulation accomplishes its intended goals of improving the quality of care and reducing the risks to clients. Studies in specific states (Applebaum and Ritchie 1992; Segal and Hwang 1994) suggest that instituting regulation on board-and-care homes drives some smaller homes out of business, increases the costs of operation for those that remain, and results in no significant improvement in the quality of care. In fact, there remain doubts about whether regulation has been effective in nursing homes in ensuring high-quality care and minimizing risks to patients (Vladek 1988).

A recent study examining the effects of licensure on larger homes in California (averaging over thirty beds per home) suggested that the major change following licensure was increased costs. There were few differences in the indicators of quality used in the research (Segal and Hwang 1994), raising questions as to its efficacy as a strategy to enhance the quality of care. Licensed homes also took a more institutional orientation toward their clientele and charged higher fees than did the unlicensed facilities, yet did not provide superior care (Segal and Hwang 1994).

Regulatory oversight intends to reduce risk by protecting against the few notorious providers who violate most reasonable rules in their provision of services. These cases both provide fodder for exposé writers and fuel public outrage. Oversight of the homes is considered the only means of reliably identifying such problems, but it may reflect a futile and costly attempt to remove all risk.

A second major question that remains is how to treat small board-and-care homes in terms of the development of regulation (e.g., as mini-institutions, as quasi-familial settings, or in some new fashion). According to Noll (1985, 9), regulation is a "uniquely American approach to the political control of market processes." Most of the current and proposed regulations have treated board-and-care homes as if they were small institutions, with requirements for staffing, fire safety, and space for each resident (GAO 1989; Reichstein and Bergofsky 1983). The regulations developed for nursing homes, by being familiar to those crafting legislation and implementing it, serve as models, regardless of their appropriateness in other settings (Baggett 1989). Seldom is the latitude given to family caregivers considered an appropriate model for board-and-care homes, since this would both admit risk and ignore the payment-for-care side of the relationship. In families, regulators rely on emotional bonds to control risk to dependents, a questionable assumption across-the-board, given our knowledge of familial abuse (Steinmetz 1988). Similar attachments in small board-and-care homes are not recognized, to the frustration of many of the operators we interviewed. The development of a distinct set of criteria for oversight in small board-and-care homes is beginning to be considered.

A third question is the effect of regulation on the supply of operators for small board-and-care homes. Regulations, such as those in most states, come at a cost of imposing bureaucratic requirements on good operators, which may significantly diminish the appeal of, and the autonomy associated with, providing care at home in a nonrationalized setting. If, in fact, one of the major motivators of operators is to provide high-quality care in a personalized fashion, without the paperwork requirements and regulatory distractions found in more-rationalized institutional settings, any movement toward more bureaucratic oversight may undermine the corps of providers or drive them underground (Applebaum and Ritchie 1992).

Finding Resources to Support Community-Based Care Options

There is no system in place to finance board-and-care services. Funding, like regulation, is piecemeal and subject to political forces. Fees for board-and-care homes come from both public programs (e.g., SSI, VA benefits, and Social Security) and private resources, such as pensions. Since the private-pay clients of board-and-care homes seem to be faring well in the better-financed homes (and in the new assisted-living facilities) (Newman 1989), our attention must be focused on the poorest individuals, generally housed in the lower-fee homes. These individuals rely on income maintenance programs, such as SSI, to purchase housing, meals, *and* services on funds barely adequate to purchase minimal housing in many locations. The political will to support increased expenditures for care and support of marginal, dependent, underclass individuals in these homes appears to be absent at this time.

Some prior research has suggested that select aspects of quality are related to the funding level of the homes (Lyon 1993; Newman 1989; Reschovsky and Ruchlin 1988). Our findings do not strongly support this contention, since funding was largely unrelated to many indicators of quality. The question remains as to how adequate resources can be channeled to small board-and-care homes to meet the expenses incurred by operators and to provide them with some reasonable income, a prerequisite for maintaining the board-and-care industry in the future.

Current proposals to substantially reform health care emphasize home- and community-based care options for medical, but not custodial, care. In an era of serious cost constraints, most proposals under discussion lack mechanisms for financing room, board, and personal care services required by so many functionally dependent individuals. The cost for the services that we desire for these populations exceeds the public will to collect additional taxes or redirect other funds to this purpose, placing those attempting to operate and regulate small board-and-care homes in a dilemma. The public clearly wants conditions improved in (and residents removed from) homes providing poor-quality care; yet no funds are available to monitor or support such homes on any routine basis. The very marginality of the residents reduces, as it does for welfare recipients and the homeless, both public and legislative support. The "otherness" of the marginal group encourages thinking about "them" as separate from the mainstream and therefore suspect.

The public's knowledge regarding these small homes has been restricted to the sensationalized, negative media reports on fraud and abuse (detailed in chap. 1). Clearly, they would see no reason to find additional funding for a care alternative perceived to be a failure. Public perceptions are based on incomplete information about the reality of board-and-care services. The absence of public support for additional funding may mean the eventual collapse of the board-and-care system, forcing society to face the problem of where to house the displaced client population. Other more-expensive forms of care, such as nursing homes, prisons, or hospitals, are concurrently under pressures to contain their costs. Failure to find the financial support for small board-and-care homes would, therefore, be a decision costly to residents, because many of them would be left without housing and care unless their health conditions deteriorated.

Small board-and-care homes lack a voice to lobby for increased funding and support at various levels of government. They are, as a grass-roots and largely unaffiliated industry, not organized in a way that encourages them to be recognized politically as a viable alternative. What appears to be essential is that society decide if board-and-care homes, as a community-based alternative to institutions, are a valuable option to sustain. Such a decision would appear unlikely in the current climate, given the consistently negative information available to the public.

Gender, Work Satisfaction, and Home Operators

It was far from surprising to find that the great majority of the operators of board-and-care homes were female. The provision of care to dependent populations, whether adult or child, has been and continues to be the domain of women (Abel and Nelson 1990). Gender norms in contemporary Western societies identify interpersonally nurturant and caregiving behaviors as part of the female spectrum of activities, both within and beyond the bounds of the family. Constructing an employment option whereby women can continue or extend their "mothering work" with dependent adults in their own households seems to be a logical outgrowth of these norms. The gratifications, too, seem to be largely interpersonal for women who could make more money in other employment. As we saw, some of the operators in our studies had always done this type of work, but not always received pay or conceived of it as "work."

Such caregiving work, sometimes requiring minimal formal training but relying on "maternal thinking" (Riddick 1983) or "mother's wit" (Diamond 1992) for guidance, has served as an employment venue for women with limited education and experience, whose likelihood of locating employment in other sectors may be severely constrained (Bartoldus, Gillery, and Sturges 1989; Burgio and Burgio 1990; Feldman 1990; Tellis-Nayak 1988).

Gender-related restrictions on employment opportunities have been part of the force driving women into such irregular economy activities.

The advanced age of the corps of female operators in both Cleveland and Baltimore raised the question of whether this group of altruistically motivated caregivers will be replaced in the future. This question points to a broader issue; will there be sufficient numbers of motivated care providers to manage the growing dependent adult populations in the future, whether the care occurs in board-and-care homes, assisted-living units, through home-care services, or in the more traditional nursing home environment?

It remains a significant and troubling possibility that younger women, with broader opportunities for employment and service and, perhaps, different values, may opt for employment in areas other than those providing care to the dependent populations in our society. Many others would argue, however, that provision of care will continue to be a positive choice made by women, since it is closely aligned with their gender role expectations as wives and mothers (Abel and Nelson 1990). It is unclear whether the opening of other employment opportunities, paired with the rising educational levels of women, will net them more equal access to opportunities in the regular economy's labor market (Sokoloff 1992).

If we adopt the argument that women do this potentially oppressive work because they lack alternatives to support themselves and their families, it would be logical to expect them to escape the work as soon as they can. If we adopt the more positive view voiced by the home operators in our studies, that work giving service to others, with its attendant interpersonal gratifications, is chosen as a labor of love, then the problem would appear to be much less pressing.

But can we rely on the gratifications from providing services to guarantee a sufficient pool of providers to dependent adults in the future? Will the lure of a labor of love be enough to meet the growing need? The answer depends, at least in part, on the work context associated with these jobs. If the care providers are able to receive the kinds of interpersonal gratifications of a job well done, the morale and retention of the caregivers should be less of a problem. The bureaucratization and rationalization of workplaces, however, threatens the opportunities to gain this type of reward (Ritzer 1993). We have already seen the reports by many board-and-care home operators of their dissatisfaction with working in nursing homes and their beliefs that inadequate care is provided there.

Should pressures to regulate other settings, such as board-and-care homes, provide similarly regimented and rationalized working environments, society may effectively undermine the very rewards that motivate board-and-care home operators to do their best. This is the very opposite of the manifest goal that regulation is intended to accomplish—quality care.

This concern reaches far beyond the walls of board-and-care homes and may represent some of the current difficulties seen in nursing homes and home health care work (Feldman 1990; Halbur and Fears 1986; IOM 1986). If these service motivations are quashed among those doing the "bed and body work" of care (Gubrium 1975), we may see the most problematic of situations—one in which only the most disadvantaged and least employable individuals are, by default, pulled into the work of providing care to dependent populations in the society.

Board-and-Care and the Assisted Living Movement

Small board-and-care homes face strong challenges from the growing movement to develop assisted living alternatives for the dependent elderly. Perhaps the vigor of this movement will bring about meaningful dialogue on the similarities among the various environments, both planned and unplanned, currently housing dependent adults. Our research suggested limited differences between the services provided in what we term board-and-care homes and the kinds of services suggested by many as appropriate for assisted living (Wilson 1993; Regnier, Hamilton, and Yatabe 1991).

A key question that remains is whether assisted living settings, with their privacy and wide range of services, will be able to meet the needs of poorer and marginalized individuals unable to finance their own care. Kane and associates (1993) seem encouraging about the prospect but suggest no mechanism to finance the higher costs that would, without doubt, be involved. Additional questions remain, however, regarding assisted living as a new and highly popular phenomenon. How will assisted living settings be staffed? How will staff deal with problem behaviors, especially of those with dementia? Will assisted living settings be regulated? Will regulation turn them into another institutionalized setting, with limited flexibility and autonomy for residents? Can we keep assisted living from becoming mini–nursing homes, where we attempt to contain costs by providing less care? Can a financing system be developed to protect against excessive profits at the expense of the care of residents? Will services be provided in a rationalized, institutional fashion or in a personalized, responsive fashion? Will any system accommodate poor or near poor residents (Kane, Wilson, and Clemmer 1993)?

The futures of the board-and-care and assisted living industries seem likely to be intertwined, with decisions in one shaping outcomes for the other. Given the rapid pace of discussion and development in the assisted living movement, such influences could be brought to bear on small board-

and-care homes very soon. One possible outcome is a two-tier system: privately funded assisted living for those who can afford such care and publicly subsidized board-and-care homes for those who cannot. This would more clearly establish small board-and-care homes as part of the welfare system, with its attendant stigma.

Conclusions and Recommendations

Small board-and-care homes exist between the worlds of home and nursing home, with strong pressures pushing on them from many sides. The "discovery" of board-and-care homes by policymakers places them in danger of extinction. In an attempt to protect the vulnerable populations housed within them, policymakers try to abolish risk through regulation. Clearly, operation of the market is not sufficient to preclude fraud and abuse in board-and-care homes. Making the assumption that regulation reduces risk and improves quality, society is on the verge of enacting regulations for smaller board-and-care homes that mirror those developed for nursing homes. These regulatory requirements cost money that will, without doubt, put many of the homes we studied out of business. Society lacks viable care alternatives for the large numbers of frail and dependent persons housed in small board-and-care homes, especially those who are poor or have incomes just above the poverty level. We must strive to understand the reality of small board-and-care homes as we move cautiously to develop policies to support and regulate them.

The issues faced by the various constituent groups interested in small board-and-care homes will be addressed in the next decade or two, possibly as an outgrowth of major health care reform (Doty 1993) or the assisted living movement. Based on the findings of our research, we offer the following recommendations to those developing policy and programmatic responses.

First, there is clearly a need for *more financial support* to enable the operators in lower-fee homes to provide the kinds of care their residents need (Stone and Newcomer 1986). Enabling them to do a better job by reimbursing them for the full range of costs associated with care would undoubtedly remove some stress from operators and reduce the amount of time now devoted to dealing with bureaucratic agencies. The operators themselves suggest only a modest fee for services (approximately $1,000 per month per resident in 1990 dollars), which would probably not be high enough to attract poorly motivated profiteers to small board-and-care homes.

Secondly, we suggest that operators and residents alike could benefit from active services providing *case management* and *advocacy for residents*. This recommendation comes with a strong qualification; mandating these services will not work without funding to expand current services. An earlier effort to improve board-and-care homes, through the expansion of the nursing home ombudsman program to cover these homes, failed for lack of funding. Few states were able to carry out this enlarged mandate, with the result that the overtaxed ombudsman system has been unable to effectively serve board-and-care homes or their residents (Stone and Newcomer 1986).

Case managers could both coordinate necessary services outside of the home and protect the rights of clientele. Individual assessments of whether the physical environment meets the resident's needs for services and safety would also allow oversight of the operators, any staff, and the physical environment.

A third recommendation is to *preserve the smaller home.* The concept of a provider taking dependent adults into her existing home for care is fundamentally different than the built environments characteristic of nursing homes or assisted living. In this "natural environment," operators have a stake in the quality of care that is embedded in the environment they share. Staffing, in contrast, brings persons to the environment in shifts to provide care. At the end of the shift, the staff person walks away from any problems that remain, an option unavailable to the operator of a small board-and-care home.

Small size also permits flexibility, personalization, and building of more direct, ongoing linkages that characterized the best of the homes we visited in both of our locations. As the twin pressures of cost-containment and quality control push care toward an assembly-line, rationalized state, it was encouraging to us to see the personalization of care achieved in the small board-and-care homes. Attention to individual detail in planning meals and outings can, for example, separate adequate care from a more personal ideal to which many in American society would readily subscribe. The rationalized, assembly-line care, in contrast, attends to whether caregiving tasks are completed but views workers as substitutable replacements for one another (Diamond 1992). Turnover in caregivers sharply curtails the potential for a caring, individualized relationship to evolve, reducing the gratifications to providers and permitting perfunctory treatment of clientele.

Movement away from this small size and coresiding operator ideal begins (inevitably, we believe) to move toward a more rationalized, institutional form of care that has clearly been rejected by public attitude in the United States and many other countries (Doty 1993; Reichstein and Bergofsky 1983; Segal and Hwang 1994). If people cannot be cared for in their own homes because of cost constraints, perhaps maintaining a homelike environment for care is the next best option (Doty 1993).

A fourth recommendation is that policymakers begin to accept the notion that *care cannot be given without some risk* to the vulnerable. Efforts to eliminate risk beg the question of whether it is possible to achieve this goal in light of the severely and multiply impaired populations housed in board-and-care homes. It is unclear whether regulation simply provides the illusion of control in caregiving systems that are, at their core, reliant on the goodwill of workers to meet the desired goals.

The great majority of the homes that we saw were of good quality without regulation. They relied upon the altruism and motivation of their operators to guarantee that the needs of residents were met and that their safety was protected. If the personnel are key to ensuring care of high quality, then all of the emphasis on physical structure and recording of routine care is misdirected. Regulations would best be directed at initial screening of operators and ongoing observation of them during interactions with their residents, rather than checking for adequate hallway width and food storage.

A final recommendation is that we *acknowledge and respect the work of caregivers*. This work is currently valued by neither adequate remuneration nor respect. Public images focus on fraud and abuse, regulators tend to assume the worst until proven otherwise, and caregiving work is viewed as an undesirable "default" for those unable to gain better employment. This respect should, of course, be shared with aides in nursing homes, hospitals, and home health care systems, where low wages and lack of recognition contribute to high turnover and worker dissatisfaction (Bowers and Becker 1992; Halbur and Fears 1986). Many of the operators we interviewed suggested that they felt unappreciated, especially when families or regulators questioned their dedication or skill.

Recruiting and retaining a cadre of highly motivated providers in this climate is constrained by the uniformly negative images presented of this type of work and the persons involved in it. We suspect that the tendency of some operators to avoid regulators and community awareness of their work (including participation in research) derives from this lack of respect and suspicion toward the kind of work they do.

Any decisions that will be made pertaining to regulation, financing, or support in small board-and-care homes will reach beyond this limited segment of the continuum of care for dependent populations. They will shape the options available for care for all of us who require some assistance at some point in our lives. Whether society is willing to assist in the financing of that care, whether that care is "professionalized," whether it is provided in centralized institutional facilities, and what groups within the population are eligible are all key questions that will have ramifications far beyond the walls of board-and-care homes.

Appendix: Details of the Research □

The information presented in this book reflects a ten-year research process in two major urban areas, Cleveland, Ohio, and Baltimore, Maryland. Details of the purposes, design, and methodology of each of the two studies, named after their cities, are provided below.

The Cleveland Study

The Cleveland study grew out of a cooperative relationship between one author (Eckert) and a community organization, the Boarding Home Advocacy Program (BHAP). This nonprofit ombudsman program was part of the statewide network to extend ombudsman services to board-and-care facilities in the five-county Cleveland metropolitan area. In the early stages of this effort, the committee realized the need for basic information on small board-and-care homes operating in the Cleveland metropolitan area.

In January 1983, Eckert, in cooperation with Sally Reisacher, who was working with BHAP, launched a six-month pilot study to obtain basic information about small board-and-care facilities and the people who lived in them in Cleveland and Cuyahoga County. The study involved in-person interviews with providers of board-and-care services to make initial observations, develop tentative general propositions, and draw conclusions that could guide further questions and observations (see Babbie 1979).

The sample of homes used in the pilot study was selected from the pool of homes identified by the BHAP of Cleveland. At the time of the survey, 275 board-and-care facilities were thought to be operating in the Cleveland metropolitan area. Forty operators who had at least one resident were interviewed for the pilot study; thus information obtained about residents was based on the operators' assessments of them. Findings of this pilot study shed new light on the operators, the residents, and the homes themselves and raised important researchable questions.

The pilot study was important to the larger study that followed in several ways. First, it solidified the working relationship with the community-based organization (BHAP) critical for identifying small board-and-care homes in the Cleveland metropolitan area. Second, the pilot study demon-

strated that operators of such facilities were accessible and willing to participate in social research. Third, it pinpointed an important question beg-
ging for answers—to what extent were these small board-and-care homes
adequately meeting the needs of the clients they served? The published
research and policy literature addressing this question was small at that
time, and the conclusions were contradictory. One problem with the existing studies was that they lumped together facilities that varied on the basis
of size, services rendered, populations served, and the levels of care required by residents.

Following the completion of the pilot study in Cleveland, a proposal to
examine the social and physical characteristics of small board-and-care
homes from the perspectives of operators and residents (i.e., the insider's
perspective) was developed and submitted to the National Institute on
Aging (NIA) and was funded in 1985. The purposes of the thirty-six-month
study "Unlicensed Board-and-Care Homes and Residents' Well-Being"
were to provide a detailed description of small board-and-care homes from
the perspectives of both their operators and their residents; examine how
characteristics of the board-and-care homes' physical and social environments affected older residents' psychosocial well-being and satisfaction;
and discover the relationship among the health status and demographic
characteristics of the residents, their satisfaction with the home, and their
psychological well-being. The study also addressed the controversy of
whether the informal organization of the board-and-care home provided
sufficient benefits to counteract the limitation in resources and formal
supports experienced by such homes.

Selecting Homes, Operators, and Residents

The research was carried out in Cleveland, Ohio, and surrounding counties, which included urban, suburban, and rural areas. The sample was
selected from two sources, BHAP records and Social Security Administration State Data Exchange (SDX) tapes. BHAP had general information on
approximately 533 homes of varying size and sponsorship (e.g., religious,
nonprofit, proprietary) in the five-county area. The list was unstable, however, since homes relocated, opened, or closed continuously. The SDX
tapes were used as a supplemental source for identifying small board-and-
care homes. The SDX tapes provided a listing of all SSI recipients (or
representative payees) by county and zip code. Residences could then be
identified where two or more checks were received, and those in which the
recipients appeared to be unrelated were assumed to be board-and-care
facilities, until proven otherwise.

By the end of May 1986, a total of 1,063 possible board-and-care homes had been identified from all sources in Cuyahoga and the five surrounding counties. Homes were eligible for the study if they housed at least one resident sixty years of age or older and contained a total population of no more than twenty-five residents. Only 16 percent of the homes on the original list were determined to be suitable for inclusion in the sample. While this percentage seemed low, it reflected a dynamic environment in which licensing and monitoring did not exist. Some homes did not have a resident at the time of contact, and others had only residents below age sixty. Some persons contacted were confused about the label "board-and-care," denying that they were providing such services. Other caregivers known to the BHAP to be active and to have residents over age sixty identified themselves as out of business, seeking, apparently, to avoid inclusion. We do not know why some operators avoided participation in the study.

The SDX tapes did not prove to be an effective tool for augmenting the sample, since only three additional homes were identified by this approach. Of the twenty-seven board-and-care homes meeting study criteria identified through analysis of the SDX tapes, twenty-four were already recorded in BHAP files. This suggested, however, that in areas without programs similar to BHAP, analysis of the SDX tapes could serve as a useful methodology for identification of small board-and-care homes. Whereas the SDX tapes may have biased the sample in the direction of low-income residents, this was not a problem, since low income is a defining characteristic of the board-and-care home population (Capitman 1989; Dittmar et al. 1983)

Efforts to identify small board-and-care homes showed that they went in and out of business without much notice. For example, dozens of homes known to BHAP to have residents during the months before the sample identification phase reported none at the time of telephone screening. Other homes changed quickly in terms of resident status. For example, one home had five residents at the time of screening and only two a few months later at the time of the interview; another had five at screening and twelve at the time of the interview. Finally, another several dozen could not be reached after repeated attempts, because phone numbers were unlisted or the phones were disconnected or changed, with no new number. In such cases, even cross-checking with address-keyed telephone books was of little assistance in making contact.

The screening process yielded 198 facilities meeting selection criteria. In an attempt to increase the number of homes and residents to be interviewed, the minimum age for residents was lowered to forty-five. This, however, yielded only a few additional homes. The final sample consisted of 177 operators, since 21 refused to participate in the study.

Of 594 residents reported by the operators as currently living in the homes, approximately one-half were interviewed. When the operators had agreed to be included in the study, they identified all residents forty-five years old and older. Operators were consulted concerning the resident's ability to respond to an interview. When the residents identified as able were approached, they were asked to be part of the study. Those who agreed to be interviewed constituted the resident sample. In most instances, interviewers made at least a second visit to each home to complete the resident interviews.

Reasons that residents were not interviewed included refusal on the part of the operator acting as a gatekeeper, refusal by the resident, judgment by the interviewer that the resident was too physically or mentally impaired, absence of the resident from the home, and failure of the resident to meet the age criterion. The final sample consisted of 285 residents. Of the residents interviewed, 273 qualified on the mental status examination for inclusion in the study and analysis, and 254 were over the age of sixty.

The primary method of data collection in the Cleveland study was structured, focused interviewing. Two separate interview schedules, combining forced-choice and open-ended questions, were used to interview operators and residents. The face-to-face interviews were conducted in the board-and-care homes between February 1986 and March 1987. Five experienced interviewers received ten hours of interview training before entering the field. The interviewers were matched by race to the respondents whenever possible.

The research team, which included the Principal Investigator (Dr. Kevin Eckert), the Co-Principal Investigators (Drs. Marie Haug and Eva Kahana), the Project Director (Dr. Kevan Namazi), and a representative from BHAP (Dr. Sally Reisacher), developed both the caregiver and resident interviews. The interview administered to the operators asked questions pertaining to the physical characteristics of the board-and-care environment, the kinds of residents the operator would accept, the rules governing residents, the records kept on the residents, the former care and living arrangements of residents, the social interactions of residents, the kinds of services supporting the operators and the residents, and the demographic and personal characteristics of the operators.

The resident interview was developed with the assistance of the project consultant, Dr. Robert Rubinstein. Separate scales were used to measure social and physical aspects of the environment, resident characteristics, social supports, recent losses, mental and physical health status, psychological well-being, and environmental satisfaction. Additional measures were developed for assessing the familial and homelike atmosphere of board-and-care residences, an area in which Dr. Rubinstein was particularly helpful. Both the provider and the resident interviews ranged from one to two hours in length.

Immediately following the data collection with the operators and the residents, the interviewers provided written comments on the physical condition of the home and the rapport during the interview. These comments, along with regular debriefing sessions between the interviewers, Principal Investigator(s), and Project Director, yielded additional qualitative information about the homes and the people who lived in them. Data from this Cleveland study serve as one of the two major sources used in this book.

The Baltimore Study

In 1987, following the move of author Eckert to Baltimore, a small pilot study was conducted replicating the data collection methods and cross-sectional design developed in Cleveland with a small ($N = 47$) convenience sample of homes in the city of Baltimore and five surrounding counties. At that time, Maryland required licensure or certification for any residence housing four or more unrelated adults. Therefore, the population of interest in the Baltimore area was defined as board-and-care homes having three or fewer residents. The pilot sample was drawn nonrandomly from a list of 225 people believed to be operators of board-and-care homes, gathered through contacts with city and county departments of health, aging, and social services and all metropolitan area hospital departments of social services. Thirty-four residents in these homes were also interviewed.

The pilot study showed that the homes in Maryland were similar in many respects to those in Ohio, except that more were located in urban, low-income areas. Also, because of variations in state regulations, the homes in Maryland had slightly fewer residents per home. Costs for care were also lower, and a higher percentage of Baltimore-area operators were African American.

While the research conducted in Ohio provided an in-depth description of the operators and the more healthy residents of small board-and-care homes, it excluded those who were more frail and unable to be interviewed. Moreover, there was a gap in our understanding of the effects that providing care to these at-risk elderly residents had on the operators. How did ongoing responsibility for multiple adults with physical, cognitive, and mental impairments affect the operators? The growing literature on caregiver burden in families added urgency to this focus.

A subsequent NIA-funded project, here referred to as the Baltimore study, improved upon two specific methodological limitations in the Cleveland study: its cross-sectional design, which provided information at only one point in time, and the collection of information on only those residents who were sufficiently mentally alert to be interviewed.

An application for continuation of the grant was written in 1988 and submitted to NIA for funding. Authors Eckert and Morgan were the Principal Investigators and Lyon served as the Project Director. In April 1989, a three-year, longitudinal, continuation project, "Caregivers to At-Risk Elderly Board-and-Care Home Residents," began. The multimethod approach included four semistructured and face-to-face interviews with caregivers, with supplemental telephone contacts between interviews; health evaluations of randomly selected older residents of homes in the sample; and qualitative observations in the homes.

The Baltimore study was designed to produce two important results. First, longitudinal data were collected from board-and-care operators concerning physical, emotional, and financial burdens experienced by them and the effects that burden had on decisions they made about the operation of the home (i.e., continuing to operate, number of residents accepted, and removal of particular residents). Nearly 100 operators of small, largely unregulated, board-and-care homes in the city of Baltimore and five surrounding counties were interviewed four times over an eighteen-month period. Given that these environments provided varying levels of care to a segment of the at-risk elderly population, the second important result of the study was a description of the objective health status of a randomly selected sample of elderly board-and-care home residents, evaluated by trained health care professionals.

Population Identification and Sample Selection

As noted earlier, a list of 225 small board-and-care homes had been generated in 1987 when the pilot study was conducted in the Baltimore area. This list was updated and expanded in 1989, using the same sources supplemented by three private referral agencies, resulting in a list of 485 potential homes. Originally, the sample selection criteria included homes that were currently operating, nonregulated, and housing at least one older (aged 60 years or above) adult. However, to enhance the sample, Project HOME residences were added with the cooperation of the Maryland Department of Human Resources.

The Project HOME Program, established in 1978, follows an integrated model (Mor, Sherwood, and Gutkin 1986) that monitors quality while providing support to home operators as well as residents of small board-and-care homes. The program includes regulations appropriate to small homes, case management for its clients, and supplementation to SSI for special rates of reimbursement. Although originally intended to serve non-elderly mentally and physically disabled persons, the program was expanded to include dependent adults of all ages. While serving a significant and growing number of older persons (in 1990, 35 percent of Project HOME clients were sixty-five years and older), a large percentage of clients in the program are younger and male, reflecting characteristics of the deinstitutionalized mentally ill population.

In early 1992, there were 1,053 Project HOME–certified beds in 448 sites with 406 care providers throughout Maryland. Beds were located in supervised apartments, group homes, and private homes (small board-and-care homes). At the time data were collected, 776 of the beds were in private homes, with a maximum of three clients in each home. It was some of these facilities that were included in the study.

Screening

Telephone calls were made to all homes on the list to screen for those that were still in operation, were not regulated by the Maryland Department of Health and Mental Hygiene or the Office on Aging, and had at least one resident over the age of sixty. This process shortened the list of eligible homes significantly. Names, addresses, telephone numbers, and other relevant information, including Project HOME participation, were entered into a computerized data base.

Telephone screening revealed 234 homes eligible to participate in the study. Of those 198 were selected through systematic random sampling from the database. Of these homes, 108 operators were successfully interviewed, 42 refused, 33 were subsequently found to be ineligible for the study, and 15 could not be contacted because of the absence of working telephone numbers or nonresponse to messages. Of those operators contacted and eligible, 72 percent were successfully interviewed during the first wave of the study ($N = 108$).

These numbers, however, were subsequently reduced by attrition. In the six months between the first two interviews, twelve operators dropped out of the study, most reporting lack of interest or time to participate or the cessation of board-and-care services. In subsequent interviews, however, one of these returned, and only three more respondents eventually dropped out of the study. The data collection component of the Baltimore study was completed between April 1989 and June 1992, with ninety-four home operators completing all four interviews (87 percent of the original sample). Comparison of the homes in Baltimore that dropped out with those that continued on twelve sociodemographic variables revealed that dropouts were likely to be somewhat more burdened, less likely to have children in the household, and more likely to be in the lowest income category at the initial interview. None of the differences, however, were statistically significant.

During the first interview, operators were asked to provide detailed information regarding up to four current clients in their homes, generating reports on 246 current residents. We asked interviewers to select older (aged sixty or above) clients in preference to younger ones when more than four residents currently lived in the home, making this sample purposely skewed toward older residents.

In subsequent interviews with the operators in Baltimore, we asked a restricted set of questions about additional individuals who had moved into the homes, either to fill existing vacancies or to replace residents who died or left the home for other reasons. The maximum number of additional residents for whom data were collected in this way was four, so overall information on residents ranged from one to eight possible per home. Most homes fell toward the lower end of this distribution, and many homes had stable resident populations during the course of our data collection. Through operators' reports, data were available on a total of 343 residents of the homes analyzed here.

For the third component of the study, an in-depth health evaluation was conducted on one older (above sixty) resident in each home. The sample was a subset of the 246 residents described above and was randomly selected. Only eighty-five such evaluations were completed, however, because of dropouts from the study after the first interview, homes that temporarily did not have an older resident, or the operator's refusal to give access, because of protectiveness toward frail older residents in their homes.

Data Collection Methods

Three methods of data collection were used in the longitudinal study in Baltimore: semistructured face-to-face interviews with operators (with bimonthly follow-up telephone contacts); health evaluations with elderly residents; and qualitative observations and interviews.

The semistructured face-to-face interviews with operators included both forced-choice and open-ended questions. To examine the impact of physical, emotional, and financial burdens on operators' decision-making processes, a caregiver burden and attitude scale was administered during each of the four face-to-face interviews with operators. Questions concerning changes in the lives of the operators and clients were asked in the second, third, and fourth interviews. Between face-to-face contacts, the interviewers telephoned the operators to track major changes for them or their residents.

In addition to the repeated questions and measures of caregiver burden and changes in the operator's or client's lives, each interview had several themes, as mentioned in chapter 1. Like the interviews with Cleveland operators, the first interview in Baltimore asked the operators questions about their background and motivations, home operations, formal and informal supports, and the clients currently residing in the home. The second interview examined physical dimensions of the housing and care environment and the economic aspects of running the home. Social interaction within the home (what we termed *familism*), the operator's attachment to clients, departures of clients, and altruism were the focus of the third interview. Finally, regulation by external authorities, rules within the home, quality, respite for the operator, and community acceptance were topics in the fourth interview.

Instrument Development

The four *semistructured interviews* incorporated both existing and new measures. A group process involving project staff, consultants, and a representative of the board-and-care community assisted in the development of the questions and scales. For example, the twenty-three-item scale used to measure caregiver burden combined questions used in prior studies with others created specifically for this population. Dr. Steven Zarit, a leading scholar in caregiver burden studies, assisted the team in developing the caregiver burden scale. Dr. Susan Sherman provided expertise in developing questions to assess the familylike characteristics of board-and-care homes. In the early phase of the research, the director of a private community-based client referral and coordination agency serving small board-and-care home operators assisted the team in formulating questions and topics for examination. Qualitative and unstructured interviews with several caregivers in Baltimore were conducted prior to the development of the first interview, to enhance cultural sensitivity.

Following the first interviews with operators, the field interviewers became an integral part of subsequent instrument development. The longitudinal design of the study allowed us to go back to respondents to clarify seemingly contradictory findings and to follow up on important new leads that emerged from earlier interviews or ethnographic observations.

The interviews were conducted by four advanced graduate students in the social sciences with degrees in social work, nursing, sociology, and psychology. During the data collection phase of the study, regular debriefing sessions were held between the project staff and the interviewers.

In these sessions, the research team discussed observations made in the field, marked progress, and solved problems encountered during the interview process. The need to explain their field and journal notes and to respond to probing questions from other interviewers and program staff resulted in greater detail and richness than could be achieved by written notes alone. Sometimes, through the process of sharing experiences and responding to questions, whole new dimensions were discovered for investigation (e.g., the altruistic motivations of operators). Several key debriefing sessions were tape recorded and transcribed, then coded by the project staff. Some of the topics and themes emerging from this process became leads to new categories for questions in subsequent interviews, while other comments assisted the project team in understanding and interpreting responses to forced-choice and open-ended questions. Team meetings between project staff and interviewers proved to be an exceedingly strong way to bring the collective strengths of the research team to bear on theoretical concerns as well as issues of practice and public policy. These sessions were critical in formulating questions for inclusion in the second, third, and fourth round of semistructured interviews with operators.

The repeated interviews built rapport between the interviewers and operators, helped to overcome responses based solely on social desirability, and concerns that we represented the "authorities." Rapport encouraged frank discussions, and in some cases, the interviewers became confidants for the operators, with periodic contacts continuing beyond the end of the study. The close relationships between interviewers and operators necessitated a process of leave-taking. All operators were given a certificate, signed by the Principal Investigator, acknowledging their participation in the study as part of that process of closure.

The *health evaluation* was noninvasive, using both questionnaire and observational data. The evaluations were conducted in the homes by trained nurses with a Master's level of education and experience in geriatrics. In those instances in which a resident was too impaired to be interviewed (e.g., scoring below sixteen on the mini-mental status examination), proxies (who in most cases were the operators) were used. Health evaluators first administered a mental status evaluation (mini-mental status examination) (Jorm et al. 1988; Uhlmann, Larson, and Bucher 1987); then checked and recorded pulse, weight, temperature, and blood pressure. This initial screening was followed by questions on doctor visits, hospital admissions, and nursing home stays; activities of daily living; a general health status evaluation; and the use of medications. For activities of daily living, the residents were asked if they could perform the activity without help, could with some help, or were completely unable to do so.

The general health status questions covered seven systems: respiratory, cardiovascular, gastrointestinal, genitourinary, musculoskeletal, neurological, and skin.

As part of the medication profile, the respondents were asked when and how each medication was taken, if they knew why each was taken, if it was taken correctly, and what problems were encountered in taking it. Additional questions were asked about problems encountered in refilling prescriptions, paying for medications, and symptoms associated with taking medications. In addition to the interview data, the nurse evaluators observed other health problems, the overall medical condition, and the mental status of the respondent. The possible effects of others present during the interview were also noted. An assessment also was made about the adequacy of the physical environment and the availability and use of assistive devices and appliances.

The *qualitative methodology* involved several techniques: observation; informal, qualitative interviewing; and collection of life history data. The qualitative and ethnographically oriented information was collected by the trained interviewers, the Principal Investigator(s), and collaborating anthropologists (Drs. Jay Sokolovsky and Maria Vesperi). Each of the Principal Investigators made informal visits to homes to talk with operators and residents. Collaborating anthropologists conducted ethnographic observations in five homes and corresponding in-depth interviews. In-depth interviews also were conducted by Dr. Derek Gill with four other operators on the economic and financial aspects of home operation. Additionally, open-ended questioning and interviewing was used to examine specific instances of operator decision making related to changes in residents' health and status.

Data Analysis

In both studies, data from the structured interviews with operators and residents (in Cleveland) and the health evaluation data (in Baltimore) were coded and entered into data files for analysis using the SPSSx statistical package. In both Cleveland and Baltimore, the information was linked, so that resident information was connected to corresponding home and operator information for purposes of analysis. In Baltimore, this entailed linking four operator interviews with the resident health evaluations.

Analysis is primarily descriptive, comparing Cleveland and Baltimore where possible, and examining several dimensions (home size, operator's race, fees above or below average, and participation in Project HOME) as appropriate to the topic. Further details on methodology are available from the authors.

References □

Abel, E. K., and M. K. Nelson. 1990. Circles of care: An introductory essay. In *Circles of care: Work and identity in women's lives*, edited by E. K. Abel and M. K. Nelson. Albany: SUNY Press.

Applebaum, R., and P. Phillips. 1990. Assuring the quality of in-home care: The 'other' challenge to long-term care. *Gerontologist* 30:444–50.

Applebaum, R., and L. Ritchie. 1992. *Adult care homes in Ohio*. Oxford, Ohio: Miami University.

Aptekar, H. H. 1965. Foster and home care for adults. In *Encyclopedia of social work*, edited by H. L. Lurie. New York: National Association of Social Workers.

Avorn, J., P. Dreyer, K. Connelly, and S. B. Soumerai. 1989. Use of psychoactive medication and the quality of care in rest homes. *New England Journal of Medicine* 320:227–32.

Babbie, E. R. 1979. *The practice of social research*. Belmont, Calif.: Wadsworth.

Baca Zinn, M. 1989. Family, race and poverty in the eighties. *Signs: Journal of Women in Culture and Society* 14:856–74.

Baggett, S. A. 1989. *Residential care for the elderly: Critical issues in public policy*. New York: Greenwood.

Bartoldus, E., B. Gillery, and P. J. Sturges. 1989. Job-related stress and coping among home-care workers with elderly people. *Health and Social Work* 14:204–10.

Belgrave, L. L., M. L. Wykle, and J. M. Choi. 1993. Health, double jeopardy, and culture: The use of institutionalization by African-Americans. *Gerontologist* 33:379–85.

Bernstein, J. 1982. Who leaves—who stays: Residency policy in housing for the elderly. *Gerontologist* 22:305–13.

Birkel, R. C., and C. J. Jones. 1989. A comparison of the caregiving networks of dependent elderly individuals who are lucid and those who are demented. *Gerontologist* 29:114–19.

Blake, R. 1987. Boarding home residents: New underclass in the mental health system. *Health and Social Work* 12:85–90.

Boldt, M. A. 1992. The impact of companion animals in later life and considerations for practice. *Journal of Applied Gerontology* 11:228–39.

Bowers, B., and M. Becker. 1992. Nurse's aides in nursing homes: The relationship between organization and quality. *Gerontologist* 32:360–66.

Bradburn, N. M. 1969. *The structure of psychological well-being.* Chicago: Aldine Publishing.

Braun, K. L., K. J. Horwitz, and J. M. Kaku. 1988. Successful foster caregivers of geriatric patients. *Health and Social Work* 13:25–34.

Brody, E. 1975. Intermediate housing for the elderly: Satisfaction of those who moved in and those who did not. *Gerontologist* 15:350–56.

Brody, E. M., P. Johnson, M. Falcomer, and A. Lany. 1983. Women's changing roles and help to the elderly: Attitudes of three generations of women. *Journal of Gerontology* 38:597–607.

Brody, E. M., M. H. Kleban, P. T. Johnsen, et al. 1987. Work status and parent care: A comparison of four groups of women. *Gerontologist* 27:201–7.

Burgio, L. D., and K. L. Burgio. 1990. Institutional staff training and management: A review of the literature and a model for geriatric, long-term-care facilities. *International Journal of Aging and Human Development* 30(4):287–302.

Butler, A., C. Oldman, and J. Greve. 1983. *Sheltered housing for the elderly: Policy, practice and the consumer.* London: George Allen and Unwin.

Capitman, J. A. 1989. Present and future roles of SSI and Medicaid in funding board and care homes. In *Preserving independence, supporting needs: The role of board and care homes,* edited by M. Moon, G. Gaberlavage, and S. J. Newman. Washington, D.C.: AARP Public Policy Institute.

Carey, A. and T. Thompson. 1980. Structured normalization: Intellectual and adaptive behavior changes. *Mental Retardation* 18:193–97.

Center for the Study of Social Policy (CSSP). 1988. *Completing the long-term care continuum: An income supplement strategy.* Washington, D.C.: CSSP.

Chandler, J. T., J. R. Rachal, and R. Kazelskis. 1986. Attitudes of long-term care nursing personnel toward the elderly. *Gerontologist* 26(5):551–55.

Chappell, N. L., and M. Novak. 1992. The role of support in alleviating stress among nursing assistants. *Gerontologist* 32(3):351–59.

Chen, A. 1989. The cost of operation in board and care homes. In *Preserving independence, supporting needs: The role of board and care homes,* edited by M. Moon, G. Gaberlavage, and S. J. Newman. Washington, D.C.: AARP Public Policy Institute.

Chenoweth, B., and B. Spencer. 1986. Dementia: The experience of family caregivers. *Gerontologist* 26(3):267–72.

Conley, R. W. 1989. Federal policies in board and care. In *Preserving independence, supporting needs: The role of board and care homes,* edited by M. Moon, G. Gaberlavage, and S. J. Newman. Washington, D.C.: AARP Public Policy Institute.

Deimling, G. T., and V. L. Smerglia. 1992. Involvement of elders in care-related decisions: A black/white comparison. *Family Relations* 41:86–90.

Diamond, T. 1990. Nursing homes as trouble. In *Circles of care: Work and identity in women's lives,* edited by E. K. Abel and M. K. Nelson. Albany: SUNY Press.

Diamond, T. 1992. *Making gray gold: Narratives of nursing home care.* Chicago: University of Chicago Press.

Dillard, B.G., and B. L. Feather. 1989. Attitudes of in-home care aides toward elderly persons: Refinement of the Oberleder Attitude Scale. *Perceptual and Motor Skills* 69:1103–6.

Dittmar, N. 1989. Facility and resident characteristics of board and care homes for the elderly. In *Preserving independence, supporting needs: The role of board and care homes,* edited by M. Moon, G. Gaberlavage, and S. J. Newman. Washington, D.C.: AARP Public Policy Institute.

Dittmar, N., and G. P. Smith. 1983. *Evaluation of board and care homes: Summary of survey procedures and findings.* Denver, Colo.: Denver Research Institute.

Dittmar, N. D., G. P. Smith, J. C. Bell, C. B. C. Jones, and D. L. Manzanares. 1983. *Board and care for elderly and mentally disabled populations: Final report.* Denver, Colo.: Denver Research Institute.

Dobkin, L. 1989. *The board and care system: A regulatory jungle.* Washington, D.C.: AARP.

Donahue, W. T., and W. E. Oriol, eds. 1981. Housing the elderly deinstitutionalized mental patient. *Psychiatric Quarterly* 55:81–224.

Doty, P. 1993. International long-term care reform: A demographic, economic, and policy overview. *Journal of Cross-Cultural Gerontology* 8:447–61.

Dougherty, C. J. 1992. Ethical values at stake in health care reform. *Journal of the American Medical Association* 268:2409–12.

Dunlop, B. D. 1979. *The growth of nursing home care.* Lexington, Mass.: Lexington Books.

Eckert, J. K. 1980. *The unseen elderly: A study of marginally subsistent hotel dwellers.* San Diego, Calif.: San Diego State University Press.

Eckert, J. K. 1987. Ethnographic research on aging. In *Qualitative gerontology,* edited by G. D. Rowles and S. Reinhart. New York: Springer.

Eckert, J. K., and S. Lyon. 1991. Regulation of board and care homes: Research to guide policy. *Journal of Aging and Social Policy* 3(3/4):147–62.

Eckert, J. K., and S. Lyon. 1992. Board and care homes: From the margins to the mainstream in the 1990s. In *In-home care for older people: Health and supportive services,* edited by M. G. Ory and A. P. Duncker. Newbury Park, Calif.: Sage.

Eckert, J. K., S. M. Lyon, and K. H. Namazi. 1990. Congruence between residents and the environment in small board and care homes. *Adult Residential Care Journal* 4:227–40.

Eckert, J. K., and M. Murrey. 1984. Alternative modes of living for the elderly: A critical review. In *Elderly people and the environment,* edited by I. Altman, M. P. Lawton, and J. F. Wohlwill. New York: Plenum.

Eckert, J. K., Namazi, K. H., and Kahana, E. 1987. Unlicensed board and care homes: An extra-familial living arrangement for the elderly. *Journal of Cross-Cultural Gerontology* 2:377–93.

Ehrlich, P. 1986. Hotels, rooming houses, shared housing, and other housing options for the marginal elderly. In *Housing an aging society: Issues, alternatives, and policy*, edited by R. J. Newcomer, M. P. Lawton, and T. O. Byerts. New York: Van Nostrand.

Enarson, E. 1990. Experts and caregivers: Perspectives on underground day care. In *Circles of care: Work and identity in women's lives*, edited by E. K. Abel and M. K. Nelson. Albany: SUNY Press.

Erikson, K. 1990. On work and alienation. In *The nature of work: Sociological perspectives*, edited by K. Erikson and S. P. Valas. New Haven: Yale University Press.

Estes, C. L. 1979. *The Aging Enterprise*. San Francisco: Jossey-Bass.

Feder, J., W. Scanlon, J. Edwards, and J. Hoffman. 1989. Board and care: Problem or solution? In *Preserving independence, supporting needs: The role of board and care homes*, edited by M. Moon, G. Gaberlavage, and S. J. Newman. Washington, D.C.: AARP Public Policy Institute.

Feldman, P. H. 1990. *Who cares for them? Workers in the home care industry*. New York: Greenwood.

Felton, B. J., S. Lehmann, and A. Adler. 1981. SRO hotels: Their viability as housing options for older citizens. In *Community housing choices for older Americans*, edited by M. P. Lawton and S. Hoover. New York: Springer.

Ferman, L. A. 1990. Participation in the irregular economy. In *The nature of work: Sociological perspectives*, edited by K. Erikson and S. P. Valas. New Haven: Yale University Press.

Folstein, M. F., S. E. Folstein, and P. R. McHugh. 1975. Mini-mental state: A practical method for grading the cognitive state of patients for the clinician. *Journal of Psychiatric Research* 12:189–98.

Friedson, E. 1990. Labors of love in theory and practice: A prospectus. In *The nature of work: Sociological perspectives*, edited by K. Erikson and S. P. Valas. New Haven: Yale University Press.

Frisoni, G. B., R. Rozzini, A. Bianchetti, and M. Trabucchi. 1993. Principal lifetime occupation and MMSE score in elderly persons. *Journal of Gerontology* 48:S310–S314.

GAO (Government Accounting Office). 1989. *Board and care: Insufficient assurances that residents' needs are identified and met*. Washington, D.C.: U.S. Government Printing Office.

GAO (Government Accounting Office). 1992. *Board and care homes: Elderly at risk from mishandled medications*. House Select Committee on Aging, HRD 92–45. Washington, D.C.: U.S. Government Printing Office.

George, L. K., and L. P. Gwyther. 1986. Caregiver well-being: A multidimensional examination of family caregivers of demented adults. *Gerontologist* 26:253–59.

Germani, G. 1980. *Marginality*. New Brunswick, N.J.: Transaction.

Glazer, N. Y. 1990. The home as workshop: Women as amateur nurses and medical care providers. *Gender and Society* 4(4):479–99.

Goffman, E. 1961. *Asylums*. Garden City, N.Y.: Anchor.

Golant, S. 1992. *Housing America's elderly: Many possibilities, few choices*. Newbury Park, Calif.: Sage.

Gubrium, J. F. 1975. *Living and dying at Murray Manor*. New York: St. Martin's.

Habenstein, R. W., C. Kiefer, and Y. Wang. 1976. *Boarding homes for the elderly: Overview and outlook*. Columbia: Center for Aging Studies, University of Missouri.

Halbur, B. T., and N. Fears. 1986. Nursing personnel turnover rates turned over: Potential positive effects on resident outcomes in nursing homes. *Gerontologist* 26:70–76.

Harmon, C. 1982. *Board and care, an old problem, a new resource for long term care*. Report from the Center for the Study of Social Policy, Washington, D.C.

Hawes, C., J. B. Wildfire, J. L. Lux, and E. Clemmer. 1993. *The regulation of board and care homes: Results of a survey in the 50 States and the District of Columbia*. Washington, D.C.: AARP Public Policy Institute.

Hayward, G. D. 1975. Home as an environmental and psychological concept. *Landscape* 20:2–9.

Health Care Investments Analysts. 1992. *Directory of retirement facilities*. Baltimore: Health Care Investments Analysts.

Hinrichson, G. A., and M. Ramirez. 1992. Black and white dementia caregivers: A comparison of their adaptation, adjustment, and service utilization. *Gerontologist* 3:375–81.

Holtz, G. A. 1982. Nurses' aides in nursing homes: Why are they satisfied? *Journal of Gerontological Nursing* 8(3):265–71.

Institute of Medicine 1986. *Improving the quality of care in nursing homes*. Washington, D.C.: Academy.

Jaffee, D. J. 1989. *Caring strangers: The sociology of intergenerational home sharing*. Greenwich, Conn.: JAI.

Jenkins, J. L. 1986. Physiological effects of petting a companion animal. *Psychological Reports* 58(1):21–22.

Johnson, C. L., and L. A. Grant. 1985. *The nursing home in American society*. Baltimore: Johns Hopkins University Press.

Jorm, A. F., R. Scott, A. S. Henderson, and D. W. K. Kay. 1988. Educational level differences on the Mini-Mental State: The role of test bias. *Psychological Medicine* 18:727–31.

Kahana, E. 1982. A congruence model of person-environment interaction. In *Aging and the environment: Theoretical approaches*, edited by M. P. Lawton, P. G. Windley, and T. O. Byerts. New York: Springer.

Kane, R., K. B. Wilson, and E. Clemmer. 1993. *Assisted living in the United States: A new paradigm for residential care for frail older persons?* Washington, D.C.: AARP.

Kane, R. A., and R. L. Kane. 1987. *Long-term care: Principles, programs, and policies.* New York: Springer.

Kane, R. A., and R. L. Kane. 1988. Long-term care: Variations on a quality assurance theme. *Inquiry* 25:132–46.

Kane, R. A., and R. L. Kane. 1990. Health care for older people: Organizational and policy issues. In *Handbook of aging and the social sciences,* edited by R. H. Binstock, and L. K. George. San Diego: Academic.

Kaye, L. W. 1986. Worker views of the intensity of affective expression during the delivery of home care services for the elderly. *Home Health Care Services Quarterly* 7(2):41–54.

Kaye, L. W., and K. Monk. 1991. *Congregate housing for the elderly: Theoretical, policy, and program perspectives.* New York: Hayworth.

Knight, R. C., W. H. Weitzer, C. M. Zimring, and H. C. Wheller. 1978. *Opportunity for control and the built environment.* Amherst, Mass.: University of Massachusetts, The Environmental Institute.

Launer, L. J., M. A. H. M. Dinkgreve, C. Jonker, C. Hooijer, and J. Lindeboom. 1993. Are age and education independent correlates of the Mini-Mental State exam performance of community-dwelling elderly? *Journal of Gerontology* 48:P271–P277.

Lawton, M. P. 1980. *Environment and aging.* Monterey, Calif.: Brooks/Cole.

Lawton, M. P. 1981. Alternative housing. *Journal of Gerontological Social Work* 3:61–80.

Liang, J. 1986. Self-reported physical health among aged adults. *Journal of Gerontology* 41:248–60.

Lyon, S. M. 1993. Impact of regulation and financing on small board and care homes in Maryland. Ph.D. diss., University of Maryland Baltimore County.

Mangum, W. B. 1985. But not in my neighborhood: Community resistance to housing for the elderly. *Journal of Housing for the Elderly* 3:101–19.

McCoin, J. M. 1983. *Adult foster homes: Their managers and residents.* New York: Human Sciences.

McCoy, J., and R. Conley. 1990. Surveying board and care homes: Issues and data collection problems. *Gerontologist* 30:147–53.

Mindel, C. H., R. Wright, and R. A. Starrett. 1986. Informal and formal health and social support systems of black and white elderly: A comparative cost approach. *Gerontologist* 26:279–85.

Mizruchi, E. H. 1987. *Regulating society: Beguines, bohemians, and other marginals.* Chicago: University of Chicago Press.

Mollica, R., and B. Ryther. 1987. *Congregate housing.* Washington, D.C.: Council of State Housing Agencies/National Association of State Units on Aging.

Mollica, R. L., R. C. Ladd, S. Dietsche, K. B. Wilson, and B. S. Ryther. 1992. *Building assisted living for the elderly into public long-term care policy: A guide for states*. Portland, Maine: Center for Vulnerable Populations: National Academy for State Health Policy and Brandeis University.

Montgomery, R. J. V., D. E. Stull, and E. F. Borgatta. 1985. Measurement and the analysis of burden. *Research on Aging* 7(1):137–52.

Moon, M. 1989. Introduction. In *Preserving independence, supporting needs: The role of board and care homes*, edited by M. Moon, G. Gaberlavage, and S. J. Newman. Washington, D.C.: AARP Public Policy Institute.

Mor, V., C. Gutkin, and D. Sherwood. 1985. The cost of residential care homes serving elderly adults. *Journal of Gerontology* 40(2):164–71.

Mor, V., S. Sherwood, and C. Gutkin. 1986. A national study of residential care for the aged. *Gerontologist* 26(4):405–17.

Morgan, L. A., J. K. Eckert, and S. M. Lyon. 1993. Social marginality: The case of small board and care homes. *Journal of Aging Studies* 7:383–94.

Morrissey, J. R. 1965. Family care for the mentally ill: A neglected therapeutic resource. *Social Services Review* 39:63–71.

Morrissey, J. R., 1982. Deinstitutionalizing the mentally ill: Process, outcomes, and new directions. In *Deviance and mental illness*, edited by W. R. Gore. Beverly Hills, Calif.: Sage.

Morycz, R. K. 1980. An exploration of senile dementia and family burden. *Clinical Social Work Journal* 8:16–27.

Murray, C. C. 1988. The small congregate home. In *Housing the very old*, edited by G. M. Guttman and N. K. Blackie. Burnaby, B.C.: Gerontological Research Center, Simon Fraser University.

Namazi, K. H., J. K. Eckert, E. Kahana, and S. M. Lyon. 1989. Psychological well-being of elderly board and care home residents. *Gerontologist* 29:511–16.

Namazi, K. H., J. K. Eckert, T. T. Rosner, and S. M. Lyon. 1991. The meaning of home for the elderly in pseudo-familial environments. *Adult Residential Care Journal* 5:81–96.

Nelson, M. K. 1990. Mothering others' children: The experiences of family day care providers. In *Circles of care: Work and identity in women's lives*, edited by E. K. Abel and M. K. Nelson. Albany: SUNY Press.

Newcomer, R. J., and L. A. Grant. 1988. *Residential care facilities: Understanding their role and improving their effectiveness*. (Policy paper no. 21[1]). San Francisco: Institute for Health and Aging, University of California, San Francisco.

Newman, S. 1989. The bounds of success: What is quality in board and care homes? In *Preserving independence, supporting needs: The role of board and care homes*, edited by M. Moon, G. Gaberlavage, and S. J. Newman. Washington, D.C.: AARP Public Policy Institute.

Newman, S. J., and C. Thompson. 1987. *Board and care homes for the elderly and chronically mentally ill: A review of the literature*. Baltimore: Institute for Policy Studies, Johns Hopkins University. Mimeographed.

Noll, R. C. 1985. *Regulatory policy and the social sciences*. Berkeley: University of California Press.

Novak, M., and C. Guest. 1989. Application of a multidimensional caregiver burden inventory. *Gerontologist* 29(6):798–803.

Oktay, J. S., and P. J. Volland. 1981. Community care program for the elderly. *Health and Social Work*. 6:41–47.

Ory, M., G. Williams, T. Franklin, M. Emr, B. Lebowitz, P. Rabins, J. Salloway, T. Sluss-Radbaugh, E. Wolff, and S. Zarit. 1985. Families, informal supports and Alzheimer's Disease. *Research on Aging* 7:623–44.

Overbo, B., M. Minkler, and P. Liljestrand. 1991. No room in the inn: The disappearance of SRO housing in the U.S. *Journal of Housing for the Elderly* 8(1):77–92.

Pearson, J., V. Sumer, and C. Nellet. 1988. Elderly psychiatric patient status and caregiver perceptions as predictors of caregiver burden. *Gerontologist* 28(1):79–83.

Poulshock, S. W., and G. T. Deimling. 1984. Families caring for elders in residence: Issues in the measurement of burden. *Journal of Gerontology* 39(2):230–39.

Regnier, V., J. Hamilton, and S. Yatabe. 1991. *Best practices in assisted living: Innovation in design, management, and finances*. Los Angeles: National Elder Care Institute on Housing and Supportive Services, Andrus Gerontology Center, University of Southern California.

Reichstein, K., and L. Bergofsky. 1983. Domiciliary care facilities for adults: An analysis of state regulations. *Research on Aging* 5(1):25–43.

Reinharz, S., and G. D. Rowles, eds. 1988. *Qualitative gerontology*. New York: Springer Publishing Co., p. 243.

Reisacher, S. 1989. Quality of care: Operation and management issues. In *Preserving independence, supporting needs: The role of board and care homes*, edited by M. Moon, G. Gaberlavage, and S. J. Newman. Washington, D.C.: AARP Public Policy Institute.

Reschovsky, J. D., and H. S. Ruchlin. 1993. Quality of board and care homes serving low-income elderly: Structural and public policy correlates. *Journal of Applied Gerontology* 2:224–45.

Reverby, S. M. 1990. The duty or right to care: Nursing and womanhood in historical perspective. In *Circles of care: Work and identity in women's lives*, edited by E. K. Abel and M. K. Nelson. Albany: SUNY Press.

Riddick, S. 1983. Maternal thinking. In *Mothering: Essays in feminist theory*, edited by Triblcot. Totowa, N.J.: Rowman and Allanheld.

Ritzer, G. 1993. *The McDonaldization of society*. Thousand Oaks, Calif.: Pine Forge Press.

Rubinstein, Robert L. 1995. Long term care in special community settings. In *Long term care*, edited by Z. Harel and R. Dunkle. New York: Springer.

Savishinsky, J. S. 1991. *The ends of time: Life and work in a nursing home*. New York: Bergin and Garvey.

Savishinsky, J. S. 1992. Intimacy, domesticity, and pet therapy with the elderly. *Social Science and Medicine* 34(12):1325–34.

Scanlon, W. J., and J. Feder. 1983. *The long-term care marketplace: An overview*. Working paper. Washington, D.C.: Urban Institute.

Schneider, E. L., and J. M. Guralnik. 1990. The aging of America: Impact on health care costs. *Journal of the American Medical Association* 263:2335–40.

Schultz, D. J. 1987. Special design considerations for Alzheimer's facilities. *Contemporary Long-Term Care* 20:48–55.

Segal, S. P., and Y. Aviram. 1978. *The mentally ill in community based sheltered care: A study of community care and social integration*. New York: Wiley Interscience.

Segal, S. P., and S. D. Hwang. 1994. Licensure of sheltered-care facilities: Does it assure quality? *Social Work* 39(1):124–31.

Sherman, S. R., and E. S. Newman. 1977. Foster-family care for the elderly in New York State. *Gerontologist* 17:513–19.

Sherman, S. R., and E. S. Newman. 1988. *Foster families for adults: A community alternative in long-term care*. New York: Columbia University Press.

Sherwood, S., D. Greer, J. Morris, and V. Mor. 1981. *An alternative to institutionalization: The Highland Heights experiment*. Cambridge Mass.: Ballinger.

Sherwood, S., V. Mor, and C. E. Gutkin. 1981. *Domiciliary care clients and the facilities in which they reside*. Boston, Mass.: Hebrew Rehabilitation Center for the Aged.

Sherwood, S., and J. N. Morris. 1983. Pennsylvania domiciliary care experiment: Impact on quality of life. *American Journal of Public Health* 73:646–63.

Sherwood, S., J. N. Morris, and C. C. Sherwood. 1986. Supportive living arrangements and their consequences. In *Housing an aging society: Issues, alternatives, and policy*, edited by R. J. Newcomer, M. P. Lawton, and T. O. Byerts. New York: Van Nostrand Reinhold.

Silverstone, B. 1978. The social, physical, and legal implications for adult foster care: A contrast with other models. In *Perspective on adult foster care*, edited by N. K. Haygood and R. E. Dunkle. Cleveland: Case Western Reserve University.

Skruch, M. K. 1993. Family-likeness in small board and care homes: The measurement and prediction of the interpersonal environment. Ph.D. diss., University of Maryland Baltimore County.

Sokoloff, N. J. 1992. *Black women and white women in the professions.* New York: Routledge.

Soldo, B. J. 1981. The living arrangements of the elderly in the near future. In *Aging: Social change,* edited by S. B. Kiesler, J. N. Morgan, and V. K. Oppenheimer. New York: Academic.

Steinmetz, S. K. 1988. *Duty bound: Elder abuse and family care.* Newbury Park, Calif.: Sage.

Stoller, E. P. 1984. Self-assessments of health by the elderly: The impact of informal assistance. *Journal of Health and Social Behavior* 25:260–70.

Stone, D. 1991. *Administrative rules for residential care facilities in Oregon.* Salem: Oregon Department of Human Resources.

Stone, R., G. L. Cafferata, and G. Sangl. 1987. Caregivers of the frail elderly: A national profile. *Gerontologist* 27:616–26.

Stone, R., and R. L. Newcomer. 1985. *Long term care of the elderly.* Beverly Hills, Calif.: Sage.

Stone, R., and R. L. Newcomer. 1986. Board and care housing and the role of state governments. In *Housing an aging society: Issues, alternatives and policy,* edited by R. J. Newcomer, M. P. Lawton, and T. O. Byerts. New York: Van Nostrand Reinhold.

Streib, G. F., W. E. Folts, and M. A. Hilker. 1984. *Old homes–new families: Shared living for the elderly.* New York: Columbia University Press.

Sussman, M. B. 1978. Family, bureaucracy and the elderly individual: An organizational/linkage perspective. In *Family, bureaucracy and the elderly,* edited by E. Shanas and M. B. Sussman. Durham, N.C.: Duke University Press.

Taeuber, C. M. 1992. *Sixty-five plus in America.* Washington, D.C.: Department of Commerce, Bureau of the Census.

Taylor, R. B., and J. B. Racino. 1991. *Life in the community: Case studies of organizations supporting people with disabilities.* Baltimore: P. H. Brookes.

Taylor, R. J., and L. M. Chatters. 1986. Patterns of informal support to elderly black adults: Family, friends and church members. *Social Work* 31:432–38.

Tellis-Nayak, V. 1988. *Nursing home exemplars of quality.* Springfield, Ill.: Charles C Thomas.

Tellis-Nayak, V., and M. Tellis-Nayak. 1989. Quality of care and the burden of two cultures: When the world of the nurse's aide enters the world of the nursing home. *Gerontologist* 29(3):307–13.

Traxler, H. 1983. Share-a-home: Economics and logistics of unrelated elderly living as a family. *Journal of Applied Gerontology* 2:61–69.

Treas, J. 1977. Family support systems for the aged: Some social and demographic considerations. *Gerontologist* 17(6):486–91.

Uhlmann, R. F., E. B. Larson, and D. M. Buchner. 1987. Correlations of Mini-Mental State and modified dementia rating scale to measures of transitional health status in dementia. *Journal of Gerontology* 42:33–36.

U.S. Bureau of the Census. 1993. *Statistical abstract of the United States*. Washington, D.C.: U.S. Government Printing Office.

U.S. House. 1989. Select Committee on Aging. Subcommittee on Health and Long-Term Care. *Board and care homes in America: A national tragedy*. No. 101–711. Washington, D.C.: U.S. Government Printing Office.

U.S. Senate. 1988. Special Committee on Aging. *Aging America: Trends and projections*. Washington, D.C.: U.S. Government Printing Office.

U.S. Senate. 1991. Special Committee on Aging. *Aging in America: Trends and projections*. Washington, D.C.: U.S. Government Printing Office.

Vesperi, M. 1983. The reluctant consumer: Nursing home residents in the post-Bergman era. In *Growing old in different societies: Cross-cultural perspectives*, edited by J. Sokolovsky. Belmont, Calif.: Wadsworth.

Vladek, B. C. 1988. Quality assurance through external controls. *Inquiry* 25:100–107.

Whorley, L. W. 1978. *Social exchange patterns in the psychiatric foster home*. Doctoral diss., School of Social Work and Community Planning, University of Maryland at Baltimore.

Wilson, K. B. 1993. Developing a viable model of assisted living. In *Advances in long-term care*, edited by P. Katz, R. L. Kane, and M. Mazey. New York: Springer.

Index □

activities, 173–80, 183; chores and
helping, 174–75; of daily living (*see*
ADLs); effects on loneliness and
boredom, 178–80; factors limiting,
173, 175; shared with operator and
kin, 4, 175–78, 192, 195
ADLs (activities of daily living), help
with, in Cleveland, 160. *See* health
status, functional, of residents
advocacy: for board-and-care homes,
200; for residents, 203–4
AIDS, 102
altruism, 86–87, 94–95, 184, 191; and
familylike characteristics, 162–63;
among nurses, 86; of operators,
114. *See also* motivations of
operators
Alzheimer's disease, 102, 117, 136,
137, 148, 195. *See also* health status,
resident cognitive impairment and
assisted living, 10–11, 202–3; access
to, for poor persons, 11, 202; amenities in, 34–35; autonomy in, 41;
challenge of, to board-and-care,
202–3; compared with small board-
and-care; homes, 10–11; costs of,
11, 202; definitions of, 11, 27, 41;
size of, 11; staffing of, 202
attachment, emotional: among residents, 166–68; of operators to residents, 168–70, 185–86, 198
attitudes: of operators, toward
money, 76–80, 191; of public, to
board-and-care, 10, 15, 199–200,
205
autonomy: and decision making, 39–
40; and payment of fees, 73–74; of
residents, 37, 40–41, 49, 145, 147,

195; of work by operators, 114,
191–92, 198–99. *See also* rules

bed and body work, 202
bedrooms, 187; personalization of,
35–36, 192; single, 36, 187
burden, caregiving, of operators, 20,
95–99, 116; change in, over time,
96–97; and choice of caregiving
work, 99, 184; explanations for low
levels of, 98–99; of family caregivers, 95; financial, 97–98, 183–
84, 203; measurement of, 96–97;
multidimensionality of, 95–98; of
paraprofessional caregivers, 95; reliability of measurement of, 97–98

caregivers, 16: family members as,
193; similarities/differences of operators and family as, 95, 99, 116;
supply of paraprofessional, 113,
191, 201, 205; tradition of women
as, 86, 184, 200; traits of successful,
110–13. *See also* operators
clients. *See* residents
closing a home, considered, 95–96
community, 24; acceptance of homes
by, 12, 47–48, 49, 205; elders living
in, 120–26, 129, 147; resident interaction in, 172–73
control. *See* autonomy
cost of care: comparison with other
settings, 10, 54–55, 59, 60–61; containment of, 1, 55, 116–17, 196,
200; effect of, on residents, 129;
resident satisfaction with, 146. *See
also* expenses of operations; fees

data collection; in Baltimore, 20–21; benefits of, to operators, 185; in Cleveland, 19–20, 207–10; content of instruments in, 210, 215–17; interviewers' roles in, 215–16; techniques used in, 210, 214–15

day-care programs: need for improved services in, 110; as support to operators, 154

deinstitutionalization, 7, 21, 117, 193; mental hospitals in, 7, 118, 120. *See also* health status, and resident mental health/illness

dementia. *See* Alzheimer's disease; health status, resident cognitive impairment and

dependent adult populations, 3, 7, 182, 184, 215; housing alternatives of, 1–2, 10, 184, 185, 196–97, 200, 202–3; needs of, 10, 12, 118, 192–93; support for funding to, 196, 199–200. *See also* cost of care, containment of; financing, public

detached attachment, 88, 95, 98–99; of day care providers, 88; of operators, 95, 98–99, 116

developmentally disabled, the, 197

diversity among homes, 5–6, 186–90 (*see also* homes, board-and-care, variations among); interrelated aspects of, 189–90

economic issues in board-and-care, 8–9, 51, 183; for-profit status, 66, 70; microeconomy of homes, 52; for operators, 51; reliance on outside income, 71

elite homes, 59, 80–82, 188–89; expenses in, 81; fees in, 81; operators of, 81–82; traits of residents in, 81; variations among, 80–81, 189

employment. *See* work

equipment, 43–44; health-related, 133; safety-related, 43; variations in, among homes, 43–44

ethnicity of operator, 6. *See also* operators, race of; residents, race of

expenses of operation, 59–66; extra, 62–64, 183; food as a component of, 61, 62; measurement bias in, 60, 64–65; monthly, 61–62 (*see also* salary of operators); overall, 64–66; and regulation, 60, 84; per resident, 62; start-up costs in, 59–60; variations in, 61, 65

familial relationships, 149, 192. *See also* familylike characteristics

families of operators, 29–31; competition from, 29, 31; support from, 29, 31, 34, 151, 156–58

families of residents, 124–25; lack of close members, 170, 193; problems with, 103, 172; as supports to operators, 151, 158–60; visits from, 170–72

familylike characteristics, 4, 6, 16, 37, 99, 150, 161, 183, 186, 192, 195; altruism of operators and, 162–63; "maternal thinking," 200; operators' perceptions of, 163–66

fees, 6, 53–57; comparison of, to those of other settings, 10, 11, 54–55, 184, 188; fair, according to operators, 80, 203; inadequacy of, 104; influence of programs on, 56; keeping residents without, 77, 84; operators' reports of, 54; quality of data on, 53, 54; techniques for setting, 55–56; variation among homes in, 54–55, 56–57; variation among residents in, 55, 56–57. *See also* income

financing, private, 57–58, 127, 149, 199

financing, public, 8–9, 51–53, 66, 126–27, 182, 184, 188: accountability for, 8, 51; erosion of entitlements, 193–94, 196, 197, 199–200; federal level, 52; and incentives for

new operators, 51; of medical care,
52; multiple responsibility for, 52,
199; need for additional, 51, 109,
199, 200, 203; and regulation, 108,
199, 203, 204; and resident impairment, 52, 129; state level, 52, 53.
See also fees; Medicaid; regulation;
SSI
food: choice in, 39–40; costs of, 61,
62; resident satisfaction with, 146.
See also meals
foster care, 16. *See* homes, board-
and-care
funding. *See* fees; financing, public

gender. *See* caregivers; operators;
residents

health care, 1; experience of operators with kin, 93; key goals of, 195;
prior employment in, by operators, 93, 115, 184; reform proposals
for, 199
health status: of elderly, 1, 129; evaluations of, in Baltimore, 20, 119,
128, 216–17; functional, of residents, 128–31 (*see also* ADLs); of
operators, 91; physical, of residents, 131–34; resident cognitive
impairment and, 119, 136–38, 173,
175; and resident medications,
134–36, 217; and resident mental
health/illness, 6–7, 119, 136–38,
169; subjective evaluations of, by
residents, 128
home size, 2, 5, 10, 19, 25–26; effects
of, 4–5, 183, 186–87; limited, advantages of, 204; maximum, 21, 26;
"mom and pop" homes, 5, 26, 183;
recordkeeping and, 76; regulations
and, 5, 26; small, definition of, 4–
5, 19
homelike qualities, 13, 161, 162, 166,
185, 192, 204. *See also* familylike
characteristics

homes, board-and-care: as businesses, operator attitudes toward,
79–80, 84–85; compared with other
settings, 10–11 (*see also* assisted living; nursing homes); controversy
surrounding, 2–3; definitions of,
1–6, 209; future of, 182, 192–203;
history of, 6–7; insider/outsider
perspectives on, 13–14; numbers
of, estimated, 4; problems of operation in, 102–3, 116; public perceptions of, 15; research on, 17–21,
207–8 (*see also* research); variations
among, 17–21 (*see also* diversity
among homes); variations by home
size, 85 (*see also* home size); within
the continuum of care, 10
household, composition of: differences by operator race, 30–31, 187;
and family members, 29–31, 183;
pets, 31
housing: modifications to structures,
27, 183; ownership of, 26; types of,
26–27. *See also* dependent adult
populations, housing alternatives
of; homes, board-and-care; long-
term care; physical environment
human services personnel, perspectives; of, 13–14

impairment. *See* health status
income: amounts, to homes, 58–59;
from board-and-care, 53–59 (*see
also* elite homes); differences in
Cleveland, 57; effects of Project
HOME on, 58–59; other source of,
to board-and-care; households, 70–
71; sources of, to residents, 57–58,
85, 126–27. *See also* fees; salary of
operators
incontinence: as a problem to operators, 137, 142; of residents, 133. *See
also* health status, physical, of
residents

institutions. *See* long-term care; nursing homes

interaction, social, 185, 188; quality of, 150

interviewers, 19, 185; assessments of operator quality by, 111, 112–13; best homes, descriptions by, 194–95; ratings of home quality by, 44–46; repeated visits by, 20–21, 116

irregular economy, 82–84, 88; essential elements of, 82; importance of, 83; problems of, 83–84; small homes as part of, 83

kin. *See* families of operators; families of residents

labors of love, 113–14, 201. *See also* motivations of operators; satisfaction of operators

long-term care, 1; continuum of, 10; environments of, 24; goals of, 24; policy for, 161; problems of, 2–3, 114–15; two-tier system of, 203; unmet needs in, 25

loss, economic. *See* profit

marginality, social, 11–13, 203; consequences of, 12, 13, 117, 182, 196; in economic status, 53, 82–85; of operators as workers, 12, 115, 189; of physical environment, 24, 25, 48–49; of related settings, 182; of relationships, 116; of residents, 12, 120, 176, 189, 194, 199 (*see also* underclass); of unaffiliated providers, 87

marital status: of operators, 90–91; of residents, 118, 124–25

meals: input into content of, 39–40; sharing of, 175

Medicaid, 8–9, 52. *See also* financing, public

medications. *See* health status, and resident medications

mental illness, 6–7, 21, 43–44, 47–48, 196, 197, 215. *See also* health status, resident mental health/illness

money, operators' attitudes toward, 76–80; ambivalence about, 77, 79; role in opening a home, 76; variations in, 77–80

money management, 71–76; assistance:—for residents, 72; —from family members, 72, 74; —from professionals, 74; —payment for, through, 73; ethical issues in, 71; family economy, 85; by operators, 74–76

motivations of operators, 16, 94–95, 201, 205; altruism, 94–95, 184 (*see also* altruism); financial, 76–80, 115–16, 184, 188; importance of, 22, 113; interpersonal, 94–95, 115–16, 149, 184, 191, 201

neighborhood. *See* community

network: of operators, 158; profile of operators' support, 151

NIMBY (not in my backyard) syndrome, 47

nursing homes, 10: characteristics of residents in, 120–26; compared with family care, 161–62, 164–65; departures of residents to, 141; health of residents in, 129; regulation of, 161–62, 198. *See also* long-term care

opening a board-and-care home. *See* starting a board-and-care home

operators: ages of, 89–90; autonomy of work of, 114–15; burden among, 20, 95–99 (*see also* burden, caregiving, of operators); centrality of role of, 22, 86, 175, 185, 192; confidence among, 112–13, 117, 184; coresidence in homes by, 5; education and training of, 86, 91, 93 (*see also* Project HOME, training for operators; training of operators); of elite homes, 81–82; employment options of, 86, 200; health of, 91; identities as, 114; implications of aging of, 16, 89, 184–85, 201; limitations among, self-awareness of, 99, 116, 186; major stressors of, 98; marital status of, 90–91; poor care by, 86, 202; power of, 17, 40, 49; prior employment of, 93 (*see also* work); problems reported by, 102–3; programs to assist, 109–10; and Project HOME, 89–90; quality of skills of, 110–13; race of, 6, 89–90, 187–88; rules applicable to, 22, 116; self-assessments by, 111, 112; self-selection of, 99, 116; sex of, 91, 200; similarity to other caregivers, 88–89, 115 (*see also* caregivers, similarities/differences of operators and family as); as societal resource, 86, 88, 113; stake of, in home, 204; tenure in board-and-care of, 91–92; traits of successful, 110–13; unmet needs of, 102–3, 104–8

patients. *See* residents
payment, methods of, 72–74; reliability of, 73; representative payee option, 72; multiple, 72–74
perspectives on board-and-care: of insiders, 15–17, 182–83; of outsiders, 13–15, 22–23, 182–83, 195. *See also* community, acceptance of homes by
pets, 31
physical environment, 11, 24–50; institutional elements of, 10, 186, 198–99, 204; problems with, 28–29; quality of, 24, 44–46, 49–50, 183, 186 (*see also* quality of care). *See also* housing; space
policy, public, 182; debates in, 182, 183; Keys Amendment, 9
pride of operators, 27–28, 36

privacy, 24, 33, 36–37, 49, 145, 147; in assisted living, 11
profit, 10, 66–69; and home size, 68; noneconomic, 70; and operator salary, 68–69; per resident, 68; size of, 66–68; variation in, 66–68, 183; vulnerability of, 69, 184, 203
Project HOME, 6, 21–22, 53, 212–13; clients of, 120; effects on resident traits, 103, 120–21, 125, 126–27, 129, 131, 134, 136, 139, 141, 143, 147; fees paid by, 55, 127; recordkeeping for, 76; subsidies to other residents, 55; training for operators, 155
protection of residents. *See* risk, management of

quality of care, 1, 145, 194–97, 208; assurance of, 194–97; difficulties in assessment of, 13, 44, 194–95, 196; fees and, 8, 45, 51, 52 ; and funding, 8, 41, 42, 44, 149, 188, 194–96, 199; interviewer ratings of, 44–45, 194; role of staff in, 151, 205; variations in, 11, 45–46, 48, 187. *See also* operators, quality of skills of; physical environment, quality of
quality of life, of residents, 150

race: and attraction to board-and-care work, 89–90; difference between operator and residents, 123, 192; lack of variation by, for operators, 188; of operators, 89–90, 187; of residents, 123–24
recordkeeping, 60, 74–75 ; consistency in, 75–76; in larger homes, 74–75, 187
regulation, 4–5, 9–10 (*see also* regulators; risk, management of); absence of, 13, 107, 149; and costs, 198, 203; effectiveness of, 9–10, 197–98; effects of, 5, 186; and financing, 108, 198, 199, 203, 204; goals of, 2–

regulation (*cont.*)
3, 183, 201–2; and institutional environments, 5, 161–62, 198; and irregular economy, 84; Keys
Amendment, 9; licensure, 107,
108, 186, 197, 198; multiple agencies for, 9–10, 107, 197; in nursing
homes, 161–62, 198; problems
with, 9–10, 103; standards for, 13,
194, 196, 198–99; state differences
in, 183; and supply of homes/
operators, 198–199 (*see also* caregivers, supply of paraprofessional)
regulators, 189; attitudes toward,
107, 108; frequency of contact with,
107; as outsiders, 2, 14, 112; problems with, 108, 110; and Project
HOME, 107–8. *See also* regulation
reimbursement. *See* financing, public
relationships between operator and
residents, 16–17, 22, 84, 88, 98–
99, 175–78, 185–86, 198. *See also*
familylike characteristics
religion: role of, for operators, 191;
support from organized, in homes,
153, 154
relocation of residents. *See* residents,
departures of
research, 14; ethnographic research
process, 17–18; limitations of current, 17; locations of, 3, 19, 207–8;
longitudinal nature of, 20–21, 214–
16; methodology of, 17–21, 207–
17; purposes of, 19, 20, 208, 211–
12
residents: ages of, 118, 120–22; behavior problems of, 47, 98, 100–
101, 103, 127, 137–38, 142–44, 148,
169, 185; closeness among, 167–68,
192; clothing for, 64, 183–84; cognitive problems of, 72, 100, 102 (*see
also* health status, resident cognitive impairment and); death of,
102, 142, 169, 181; departures of,
141–45; educational achievement

of, 125–26; family (*see* families of
residents); income of, 126–27 (*see
also* income, sources of, to residents); length of stay of, 140–41,
185; marital status of, 118, 124–25;
numbers of (*see* home size); perspectives of, 16, 145–47; poverty
of, 56, 126; previous residence
of, 139–40; problematic physical
problems of, 101–2 (*see also* health
status, physical, of residents);
problems among, in locating a
board-and-care home, 17, 105; race
of, 123–24; satisfaction with care
among, 185; satisfaction with home
of, 145–47; sex of, 118, 122–23;
types of, unacceptable to operators, 99–102, 116, 184; variations
across homes, 188; work history
of, 125–26
respite: availability of providers for,
106; bartering relationships in, 106;
costs of, 106–7; duration of, 106;
and incontinence, 106–7; as a
problem, 105–6; reasons for use of,
106; unmet need for, 103, 104
risk, management of, 24, 25, 36, 86,
196, 197, 198, 203; appropriateness
of placement, 127–28; and exiting
the facility, 131; role of caregivers
in, 205. *See also* safety
rules: of behavior, 10, 37–39, 49; regarding use of space, 36–37

safety, 24, 25, 127, 147. *See also* risk,
management of
salary of operators, 60, 65, 115, 183;
and benefits, 65, 115, 183; effect of,
on profits, 68–69; Project HOME
fees as, 65–66. *See also* expenses of
operation
sample: attrition in, 21, 215–16; bias,
in residents, 119, 128; bias due to
refusal, 50, 116, 194, 210; pilot
study, 207, 211; procedures to se-

lect, 19, 208–10, 212–14; size of, 5, 209–10, 212, 215
satisfaction of operators, 69, 113–15, 191, 201. *See also* labors of love; motivations of operators
satisfaction of residents, 145–47, 185
services: availability of, in various homes, 13, 42–43, 183, 196; consistency of, across homes, 41–43, 190–91, 196; demand for, 3; funding of, 8; medically oriented, 12, 164–65; range of, 41–43, 188; unscheduled assistance, 41, 183, 190, 195
sheltered housing. *See* homes, board-and-care, definitions of
smoking: and resident health, 131; rules regarding, 38
space, 24, 25, 33–37; access to particular rooms, 34–35; problems with, 34; sharing of, 33, 48–49, 183; variation in use of, by race, 187
SSI (Supplemental Security Income), 8, 21, 51, 53, 58, 85, 184, 199, 213. *See also* Project HOME; residents, income of
staff, paid, 5, 31–33, 156, 186; in Cleveland homes, 160
starting a board-and-care home, 92–94; prior work experience and, 92–93; roles of kin and friends in, 92–93
stress. *See* burden
subsidies. *See* financing, public; Project HOME
support to operators, 150–61, 185; family members as, 156–58; formal, 150–56; inadequacy of, 104; informal, 150, 156–61; informality of, 93–94, 200; needed currently, 104, 109; Project HOME as, 155;

residents' family as, 158–60; unmet need for, 104; variability of, 93

training of operators: health-related, 134; provided by Project HOME, 155. *See* operators, education and training of

unaffiliated providers of care, 87–88; day-care providers as, 87–88; and irregular economy, 88, 201; nurses as, 87; problems of, 87–88; and social marginality, 87–88; traits of, 87; wardens as, 87
underclass: characteristics of residents, 7, 51, 199; operators as, of workers, 89

vacancies: duration of, 105; frequency of, 26, 105; filling: —need for help in, 109; —reasons for, 105; —tactics for, 104–5

welfare, 203. *See also* dependent adult populations; financing, public; SSI
work: alienation from, 114–15; dissatisfaction with prior, among operators, 115; employers' control of, 114; history of residents', 125–26; "McDonaldizing" of, 114–15; "mothering work," 200; negative attitudes toward, 113, 201; in nonrationalized settings, 115, 184; of operators outside the home, 71, 92; oppressiveness of, 61, 69, 86, 201; prior, of operators, 93; rationalization of, 114, 115, 201, 204; rewards of, 113; voluntary, by operator, 61, 69. *See also* labors of love

Library of Congress Cataloging-in-Publication Data

Morgan, Leslie A.
    Small board-and-care homes : residential care in transition /
  Leslie A. Morgan, J. Kevin Eckert, and Stephanie M. Lyon.
        p. cm.
    Includes bibliographical references and index.
    ISBN 0-8018-4996-9 (hc : alk. paper)
    1. Aged—Long-term care—United States.   2. Aged—Home care—
  United States.   I. Eckert, J. Kevin.   II. Lyon, Stephanie M.
    [DNLM: 1. Long-Term Care.   2. Homes for the Aged—United States.
  3. Home Care Services—United States.   WT 30 M848s 1995]
  RC954.4.M67   1995
  362.1'9897—dc20
  DNLM/DLC
  for Library of Congress   94-38059